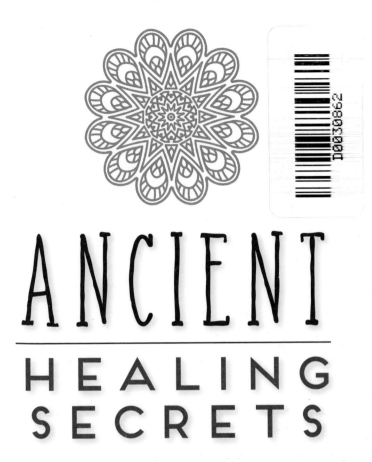

ANCIENT

HEALING
SECRETS

Publications International, Ltd.

TABLE OF CONTENTS

INTRODUCTION

How old is medicine? This is a very difficult question to answer. All living creatures have an instinct for self-preservation and take specific steps to treat themselves when their lives are threatened by injury or disease. Among many species, there is a propensity to care for one another in a family or social group: Primates groom one another; cats lick each other's wounds. This seems to be a step above self-preservation, and we might call these behaviors primitive healing. But when does an instinctual health-promoting activity rise to the level of *healing*?

One crucial factor that seems to set healing apart from self-preservation is the element of caring. An individual caring about the health of another and acting to improve it is different from merely trying to keep oneself alive. Healing is a selfless activity—an act of charity and compassion. Indeed, Buddhist medicine explicitly names compassion as the most fundamental aspect of medicine.

One uniquely human trait (arguably our defining trait, for good or bad) is our ability to, and propensity for, theorizing. Healing and health have certainly had their share of theories. Anatomy, diagnostics, therapeutics, and in some cases cosmology and theology—these theories form a medical system. Not all of the traditions we will explore had codified systems, but all had their theories—some written in great treatises, some passed down orally, and some merely outgrowths of everyday experience—that were the underpinnings of the practical craft of healing.

By this definition, the first time someone brought cool water to a feverish child because she thought it would cool the heat, medicine was born. But can you imagine a time when this would not have been the case? It doesn't even make sense to ask about a mythical first time. So, how old is medicine? It's as old as we are—probably even older.

THE TRADITIONS

Through these untold millennia, people have approached issues of health, illness, and healing in remarkably diverse ways. Despite the common goal of health and longevity, cultures around the world and through time have shown that the paths toward that goal are many and varied. In this book, we will explore some of the most intriguing traditions from around the globe. Some are the ancient roots of systems that persist today. Some are now extinct because the civilizations that practiced them died out or were wiped out. However, each displays a unique approach to the concern for health humans of every generation have always had in common.

The Near East. Through archaeologic evidence and the existence of written texts dating back to that period, we can glean a pretty good picture of how the ancient Mesopotamians of the Tigris and Euphrates river valley and the ancient Egyptians of the Nile River valley approached medicine some 3,000 years ago.

The Americas. Before the arrival of the Europeans, the Americas were not by any means "primitive" despite what the invading Europeans thought. Even today, we have trouble comprehending the healing practices of the early indigenous Americans; they are so rooted in a particular worldview, it baffles the modern Western mind. Here we first encounter shamanism, a healing system so connected with every aspect of the religion, culture, and lifestyle of Native Americans it is almost impossible to talk about it as a practice separate from any other part of life. In the Americas, we also confront the three great pre-Columbian civilizations of Latin America: the Aztec, the Inca, and the Maya. Although hampered by the deep misunderstandings of the invading Spanish, from whom most of our information comes, we get a glimpse of their advanced botanical therapeutics and surgical techniques.

Asia. Perhaps one of the oldest and richest traditions of medicine can be found in South Asia. Here, in present day India and Pakistan, the venerable science of Ayurveda was born. Springing from a synthesis of various religious and secular traditions, Ayurveda is probably the most thoroughly structured and empirically rigorous of the ancient systems. Yet its apparent complexity does not detract from its elegance or its endurance—Ayurveda is very much practiced and admired today. Yoga—in many ways a cousin of Ayurveda—also has diverse and ancient roots on the subcontinent. Japanese medicine's continuing development demonstrates how East Asia's ancient contributions to medicine remain far from obsolete.

Africa. Although the healing practices of Sub-Saharan Africa have perhaps the least archaeologic and historical information of any of the regions we explore, it is the place that has the longest history of healing in the world. Fortunately, traditions live on in modern practitioners all across the region.

THE LESSONS

Why do we care about the way medicine was practiced long ago? After all, we've made our improvements and no longer need the misguided notions and superstitions of the past. There are a number of reasons: First, the resurgence of so-called alternative medicine has fueled much controversy. Understanding the traditional basis of these approaches—from the theory of specific treatments such as acupuncture to the history and efficacy of more generalized therapies such as mind/body medicine—will allow a more thorough evaluation of their potential.

Second, the history of healing is not just a history of medicine. Healing is a social act, one that helps to define a society; the interaction between the sick and the healthy can reveal a great deal about what a culture values most. It's no accident that religion has almost always been an integral part of healing. Both are expressions of what a culture values in the face of mortality; both show what matters and what a society *does* when the chips are down. Our culture is no different, and we can use the same criteria to judge ourselves and our "superior" reasoning.

You'll find that many of the ancient ways of thinking about illness seem completely absurd. The theory that a disease could be caused by invisible demons seems to be the height of foolishness. And as for blaming ancestors for sickness—a prevalent idea in ancient times from China to the Americas—well, that one fares even worse than the demon idea.

But how different is our medicine from these ancient notions? Are microorganisms any more real to us than spirits were to them? What is the practical difference between bacteria visible only to a scientist with a powerful microscope and spirits visible only to a shaman with the proper drum? Are genetic and hereditary explanations for diseases so different or more understandable than the theories of the ancient ancestor worshipers?

There is a difference, of course. Treating dysentery as an infectious disease caused by a microorganism is much more effective than going the amulet route. Fewer people die. Insulin injections are, without a doubt, a better way to handle diabetes than trying to propitiate an offended ancestor; people live longer and with fewer debilitating complications. And the list goes on: antibiotics, angioplasty, dialysis—these scientific advances save and improve lives.

At the same time, modern Western medicine's successes and advanced methods in no way diminish the power, elegance, and, in some cases, beauty of ancient healing traditions. (Despite the computer-aided color enhancement, does a magnetic resonance image even compare to a Navajo sand painting?) And all too frequently, modernization has meant the abandonment of valuable aspects of the *art of healing* in favor of progress in the *science of medicine*.

In some respects, we've sacrificed a great deal in the name of longevity, forestalling the inevitable by making treatments more drastic and invasive. In just a few decades, we've seen the virtual eradication of monstrous menaces such as smallpox and polio, only to see the new ones such as cancer and heart disease line up to take their place. Despite our great leaps forward (and they have been great), we ultimately stand as helpless as ever in the face of death. So rather than look with disdain on the misguided ways of past generations, try to put aside your modern bias and see what you can learn from the ever-hopeful ancient healers.

SUB-SAHARAN AFRICA

The antiquity of African ideas about health, disease, and healing takes us further back in history than anywhere else in the world—back toward the very origins of humanity. The teachings and traditions of Africa's ancient hunter-gatherers reflect a deep history, going back hundreds of thousands of years.

However, this very distance in time and culture is what makes these practices difficult to discern. So the medicine from Sub-Saharan Africa (the region of Africa south of the Sahara Desert) that we will examine will be the traditional healing we see today in the region. There is reason to believe that these modern traditional practices have roots in the way of life that began around 4,000 years ago and spread throughout the continent. The truly remarkable practices of Sub-Saharan healers have a great deal in common with traditions found a world away. Aspects of shamanism, herbalism, divination, and community healing can all be found in the traditional diagnostics and therapeutics of this vast and varied region.

MAINTAINING A DISTINCTIVE CHARACTER

The Sahara Desert was not always the barrier it is now. As recently as 3,000 years ago, this region featured lush grasses and teeming herds of wildlife. Even as the rains diminished and the great desert formed, camels allowed long-distance trade between the people who withdrew southward and those who moved toward the Mediterranean. This ancient communication is why many ideas of health and healing in the Sub-Saharan region resonate with those of civilizations in the Mediterranean, the Near East, and Asia.

The medicine of ancient Egypt, for example, had significant influence in shaping the ideas of civilizations around it, including the medicine of classical Greece and Rome. Their ideas on medicine spread abroad to other African regions, especially through the influence of Islamic medicine and Galenic medicine (the medicine of humors associated with the Greco-Roman physician Galen). Christian faith healing also spread into Africa, first across North Africa and Ethiopia, then later with European influence to Sub-Saharan Africa.

Despite the commonalities African medicine has with other traditions and despite the influx of influence from elsewhere, Sub-Saharan African medicine maintains a distinctiveness. The application of these foreign ideas to the particular climates and diseases of Sub-Saharan Africa reflects the social patterns and technologic developments unique to Africa.

ANCIENT ROOTS, MODERN BRANCHES

It is likely that some of the features of current Sub-Saharan healing are adaptations of ancient hunting and gathering practices that were retained. For example, until recently, most healers collected their medicinal plants from the wild, assembling medicines fresh for each case. Now, however, some enterprising healers incorporate the cultivation of medicinal plants into their practice. Modern scientific analysis of medicinal plants in Sub-Saharan Africa continues to yield an understanding of the applications and effects of its ancient materia medica.

In West Africa, the domestication of plants and animals in sedentary settlements—as opposed to nomadic hunter-gatherer societies—was well underway by 2000 BC, giving rise to numerous local healing traditions. Urban centers emerged in the savanna by the first few centuries AD. Along with the stable settlements came trade routes that linked West Africa with the Mediterranean and Europe.

Food production and ironworking spread through Sub-Saharan Africa during the first millennium AD. Because of common cultural backgrounds, many health-related terms and concepts appear to be comparable within the region. Ecologic settings have shaped many of the ideas and practices in African healing. Depending on the ecology of an area, residents had two main options for their livelihood: cultivating crops (agriculture) or raising livestock (pastoralism). These two modes of livelihood can be practiced together in areas that have adequate rainfall for crops and the absence of certain diseases that can wreak havoc on livestock; however, these conditions are not present everywhere in equatorial Africa. Sleeping sickness (trypanosomiasis) carried by the presence of the tsetse fly was especially devastating to cattle. Throughout the forest region of equatorial Africa and parts of West Africa, the menace of the tsetse fly prohibited pastoralism. Where the tsetse fly was absent, pastoralism conveyed a distinctive set of ideas about health, sickness, and medicine. For example, in the lake regions where the agricultural and pastoral traditions overlap, nearly as many medicinal plants are used for animal husbandry purposes as for human healing. Similarly, other environmental zones of desert, tropical rain forest, and savanna have exerted their influences on health and healing. In many markets of West and Central Africa, sections are devoted to the medical plants of the rain forest on the one hand and to the arid regions on the other.

Over the centuries, the development of cultural traditions in response to ecologic settings and conditions has slowly but surely created distinctive emphases within the core of medical ideas and practices. These patterns have also determined how the medical traditions from the Mediterranean North, the Islamic East, and the Christianized and scientized West would later be received.

A COMMON CORE OF IDEAS

Across the vast area of Sub-Saharan Africa, there are, of course, many diverse healing traditions. Despite differences, however, understandings of health, sickness, and healing are often couched in a basic set of ideas about the nature of the world.

The first example of an organizing idea enveloping health, sickness, and healing defines health as the ideal, ordered structure of the body as a whole. Any disruption, negation, or distortion of this ideal suggests sickness. This idea is often expressed through the use of colors: In the Yoruba medicine of Nigeria, for example, the color of chalk (white) represents purity and wholeness; red (such as blood or the appearance of redness on the skin surface) represents transition and danger; and charcoal (black) represents human chaos. This expression of order and chaos in health and disease through a kind of color code is very widespread. It appears again and again in connection with sickness, healing, and the order of the human and natural universe.

The second idea that organizes thoughts and actions of health and healing is based on balance, or harmony. Balance is thought to be necessary in the relationship between an individual and the surrounding community, as well as between the community and the natural and spiritual environment. One of the terms expressing this sense of balance or harmony in life is *lunga*. Appearing in the vocabulary of the Zulu of southern Africa and also in the vocabulary of the Kongo of Central Africa, *lunga* is also used as an attribute of God. Indeed, the idea of balance as health and imbalance as illness is not limited to Africa. The balance between the humors and natural elements in ancient Greek medicine, the doshas in Ayurveda, yin and yang in Chinese medicine, and even the concept of *hozho* in Navajo healing testify to this concept's virtual universality.

The idea of balance is a profoundly ancient African idea expressed in many origin stories across western, central, and southern regions. In ancient creation myths, you can see how the very beginning of the world depended on the balance between the two opposing forces: In the beginning, these stories recount, a sky force and an earth force existed. (Usually the sky force was male, and the earth force was female.) A bolt of lightning or a stormy wind generated the movement to bring the two together. Out of this encounter came the combination of heat and coolness and the rhythm of light and darkness. Light and heat are found in the characters of the sun, the moon, and the stars; the earth is identified with moisture and coolness. From the encounter of these opposing spheres and forces—sky and earth, hot and cold, male and female, dry and moist—emerged the reproductive potential of the world and its creatures, bringing life into being. And the health of this life depends on maintaining the balance of the two.

HEALTH AS COOLNESS, DISEASE AS HEAT

The thermal concept of health and ill health is also widespread in Sub-Saharan African thinking. "Coolness" is grace, style, and health; "heat" is conflict and disease. (This notion of the "cool" is one of the most prominent features of African culture brought to the New World and infused directly into popular culture in North America.) In curing techniques, the heat of conflict-caused disease is "cooled down" through herbal baths and rituals.

HEALTH AS PURITY, DISEASE AS POLLUTION

Another idea used in the organization of health and disease may be expressed as purity and pollution. Purity is a ritual state in which the human world is in order. Pollution is an impersonal condition that can be righted by ritual or curative intervention. There is some similarity between this notion and the first mentioned above—order versus disruption. Purity and pollution represent a traditional set of natural contrasts that may have served as a foundation for understanding health and the prevention of disease.

HEALTH AS FLOW, DISEASE AS BLOCKAGE

The concept of flow and blockage is the closest to a classical African anatomy. Furthermore, health as flow and disease as blockage has clear implications for therapeutic practices. The prevalence of purgatives and emetics, fertility medicines, and herbal drinks in the African tool kit reflect this conceptual scheme. However, what flows and what is blocked are not necessarily the physiologic structures we might imagine; they are usually linked to the wider world of a person's relationships in society, if not to society itself as a body.

In fact, there seems to be a clear analogy between the physical realm of the body and exchanges in society. Both are seen as needing to flow openly to live and thrive. Just as food and fluids need to be taken in and ingested for the physical body to be healthy, the social body needs to be "fed" with reciprocal gifts and gestures of goodwill. Grudges, envy, and ill will in the social body are, in this thinking, seen to cause blockage in the physical body. In Rwanda, for example, one observer suggests that flow and blockage is a metaphor in which flow within the social and physical body contribute to health, whereas blockage—through envy and ill-will—may lead to constipation, infertility, witchcraft, and disease.

The principles of health and disease just enumerated—harmony versus disharmony, coolness versus heat, flow versus blockage, and so on—were used to base many of the practical diagnoses and treatments in a whole host of ailments: broken bones, fever, rheumatism, intestinal disorders, parasites, lactation deficiency, earache, toothache, headache, epilepsy, menstrual disorders, and more. Medications were based on a wide array of mineral, animal, and especially vegetable substances reflecting the desert, savanna, and forest ecologies.

A few examples illustrate the ways in which these higher-level principles were often combined to organize practical insights into treatment techniques and the curative powers of plants. Although modern Westerners will probably recognize the matter-of-fact treatment of herbal medications in the following examples, classical African medical thought often added dimensions that Westerners might call "symbolic" or "social." In the two examples of treatment by modern healers using traditional techniques, the fusion of the natural and the human dimensions is evident.

TWO TYPES OF BODILY SWELLING

Mama Mankomba of Mbemba village in the Luozi region of what is now the Democratic Republic of Congo (formerly Zaire), was well known for her treatment for bodily swelling. She distinguished between two types of swelling: One was thought to be caused by heart congestion; the other was thought to be caused by "poisoning," the result of anger growing out of the animosity of one individual for another.

Simple swelling was dealt with by an initial emetic from the drops of sap of the finger cactus (*Euphorbia tirucalli*) with a soapy base to keep the toxic sap from harming the body. This was followed by a potion made from the roots of six savanna plants taken three times daily: *Psorospermum febrifugum, Annona arenaria* (a relative of the custard apple), *Crossopteryx febrifuga* (a member of the madder family), *Syzygium guineense* (a member of the myrtle family), *Hymenocardia acida*, and *Maprounea africana* (members of the spurge family). Dietary restrictions against sugar, salt, and pepper were also imposed. Poisoning cases received the same initial purge, but were followed by a second purge of the bark scrapings of only the *Maprounea africana* plant with salt and palm oil to provoke diarrhea and vomiting.

Another example is the specific treatment for madness (*lauka* in the KiKongo language of western Congo), which was part of Kongo healer Bilumbu's longer regimen; it is the sedative for an episode of psychotic agitation. The medicinal portion of the sedative consisted of an extract prepared from the foliage of four plants: *Brillantaisia patula* (called *lemba-lemba*, a member of the acanthus family), *Virectaria multiflora* (called *kilembe-lembe kia mbwaki*, a member of the madder family), *Erigeron floribundus* (called *kilembe-lembe kia mpembe*, a relative of horseweed and part of the Compositeae family), and *Piper umbellatum* (called *lemba ntoko*, a member of the pepper family). The extract, probably thinned with water, was administered orally several times per day to assure sedation, but according to the healer, it should not be continued indefinitely because of the danger of "intoxication." (Incidentally, in a field study, this cure was clinically confirmed to be very effective.)

However, there is more to this treatment than herbs; its symbolic superstructure is intriguing. The indigenous names for all four plants bear the word *lemba* or *lembe*, which means "to calm" or "to cool." Furthermore, the part of the landscape from which these plants are gathered is important: *Lemba-lemba* grows in the domestic realm of the village; *lemba-ntoko* comes from the wild realm; and the two remaining plants—one "red" and the other "white"—originate in the gardens. The cure then suggests the sufferer's wild behavior is being domesticated or calmed.

At the chemical level, the "white" garden plant, *kilembelembe kia mpembe* (*Erigeron floribundus*) has been discovered to contain volatile oils and alkaloids that may have psychoactive and analgesic properties. The symbolic and social dimensions in this treatment include extensive support by kin and healer, analysis of dreams, and a culminating "banquet," which features the successful reentry of the sufferer back into public life and normalcy. So the cure for madness in this case combines social therapy, four symbolically charged plants, and a clinically demonstrated sedative. Which, then, is the "active" ingredient?

CURES THAT WORK

Several researchers have examined traditional African cures and found that many have merit and can be shown clinically effective. One such cure is a treatment for intestinal microorganisms practiced by Mirau, an herbalist of the Meru people. One of Mirau's 200 single-plant treatments is for children's diarrhea—a serious problem in many regions of the continent where infant mortality reaches more than 100 per 1,000 births. Using the plant known locally as *mamiso* (*Bidens pilosa*, a relative of the beggar tick), Mirau takes 15 to 20 flowers and boils them to obtain one dose, which is given twice daily as oral medicine. Although not necessarily known to the healer, this plant actually carries antibacterial substances (some unknown to Western science) against microorganisms, including five organisms that cause gastroenteritis. The same plant is used against dysentery and colic in other regions of eastern and southern Africa.

In another well-documented and researched study from the National Zairian Research Institute, the work of six healers in Kinshasa was examined for effectiveness in 22 diabetes cases. Independent examination of blood sugar levels revealed that after treatment, which lasted a week or longer, 17 of the cases experienced a significant decline in average blood sugar levels. Although a surprisingly large diversity of plants was used in preparation of the oral medications, several plants stand out for their repetition from healer to healer, including *Crossopteryx febrifuga*, *Nauclea latifolia* (both members of the madder family, Rubiaceae), *Anchonames difformis* (from the Arceae family), and *Bridelia feruginea* (from the Euphorbiaceae family), the latter of which is also used in Ghana for diabetes therapy. Some of the Kinshasa treatments were accompanied by dietary prohibitions against salt, ripe mangoes, pepper, beer, manioc (cassava), and mushrooms.

PUBLIC HEALTH AND PREVENTING DISEASE

Although very little is known about how ancient African peoples perceived the health of their communities and how they dealt with disease, some inferences suggest an approach to what we today term "public health." In some cases, the ancient practices still survive and provide clues to early concerns.

EPIDEMICS

With the transition to cultivation and larger, sedentary communities—first in the Sudan then across the continent—major new diseases made their appearance. We have some evidence of public health techniques that must have existed in ancient times in response to at least three diseases: sleeping sickness, malaria, and smallpox.

Some examples are straightforward: Hunter-gatherers, such as the Khoisan speakers of southern Africa, were known to pick up camp whenever diseases broke out or when there were deaths in a settlement. Given the small population concentrations, leaving ensured contagious diseases did not have a chance to take hold. But some public health problems were more difficult.

Livestock herding spread southward about 6,000 years ago, skirting the rain forest area. This boundary coincided with the boundary between two very different food production systems: On the one hand, the cultivators without large livestock had to emphasize crop fertility, soil fallowing, and the importance of rainfall; the pastoral cultures, on the other hand, had to manage their herds, concentrate on good breeding, and learn the politics of being good neighbors while on their annual treks to find seasonal pasture lands. But they also had to understand where the danger zones were—the habitat of the sleeping sickness-causing tsetse fly—lest they loose their cattle and their food supply.

Another insect-borne scourge native to the area was the variety of malaria carried by the anopheles mosquito. It is known to have become a problem for certain African cultivators about the time sedentary communities appeared and the forest began to be cleared for crops. One response was to avoid the mosquitoes. Breezy hillsides rather than the mosquito-infested quiet thickets are known to have been preferred sites for villages and towns (doubly so in areas inhabited by the tsetse fly). Thus, long before quinine and the association of mosquitoes with malaria, breezy hilltops were preferred settlement sites, provided they were near sources of good water.

Smallpox has been a widespread scourge not only in Africa but in the Old World ever since large concentrations of people began settling together. The earliest appearance of smallpox in Sub-Saharan Africa is not known, but Ipoona—the god of smallpox—is a central figure in West African religious beliefs, suggesting that smallpox has a history of millennia rather than centuries.

Sub-Saharan peoples took several approaches to smallpox. Sacrifices were made to the angry god Ipoona, who had the power to kill. But actions of another sort during smallpox epidemics suggest an acute public health consciousness. Reports from both West and East Africa mention the separate burial of victims, the abstinence from mourning in close proximity to the victims' bodies, and the quarantine of entire infected households or settlements.

Perhaps the most intriguing response to smallpox was the attempt to immunize those not yet infected by taking puss from the poxes of infected individuals and introducing it into scratches in their skin. However, despite the similarities to modern immunization, this ancient technique probably had less to do with inducing an immune response and more with a broader symbolic principle of confronting the evil of the disease or threat head-on.

The manner in which some other health threats were dealt with resembled the approach to smallpox. Several kinds of poisonous vipers have for ages posed a serious problem in the lands of the Nyamwezi and Sukuma peoples of western Tanzania. Organizations of snake-handling experts actively promote the encounter with these poisonous vipers and other snakes through public dance performances in which they demonstrate that they can come to terms with the threat. The demonstration includes allowing the otherwise venomous snakes to bite them.

However, the snake handlers are immune to the venom because they have been inoculated with small doses that they milked from the vipers. This understanding of immunization is a closely guarded secret available only to those who have been appropriately initiated to the Snake Handling Order. In its organization, the snake-handling fraternities resemble the *ngoma* "drums of affliction" made up of the commonly afflicted—in this case those bitten by dangerous snakes who survived.

These examples of immunization to smallpox and snake venom are part of the much wider notion across ancient Africa of the need to incorporate or confront the disease to overcome it. Snake-handling *ngoma* members sing to the spirits of the vipers to placate them and to stay in touch with them. This is not unlike the manner in which people placate with song and dance ancestral spirits that visit the living in dreams or through misfortune—public spectacle for public health.

MESOPOTAMIA

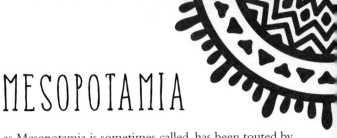

The Fertile Crescent, as Mesopotamia is sometimes called, has been touted by some to be the location of the Garden of Eden and the birthplace of humanity. Although the truth of these assertions will probably never be known, it is true that the ancient civilizations of this region were extraordinary in their culture and accomplishments.

The ancient lands of Mesopotamia lay between the Tigris and the Euphrates rivers, in part of modern-day Iraq. In fact, the name Mesopotamia means the land between the rivers. Although their flooding was violent and unpredictable, these two rivers allowed civilizations to grow and flourish, bringing with them all we think of when we use the term *civilization*—cities, monumental architecture, agriculture, the division of labor, art, government, and writing.

CUNEIFORM

Writing probably originated in Mesopotamia, with Egypt developing its own system around the same time or slightly later. About 3100 BC, the people of Sumer (Sumerians) began using pictographs—pictures representing or expressing an idea—to list livestock and agricultural equipment, probably as a business record of some kind. Using a reed, they wrote on damp clay and then let the clay dry and harden. Eventually the pictographs developed into cuneiform writing, done with a wedge-shaped reed. The Sumerians used over 600 symbols to represent the syllables of their spoken language. Because each sign stood for a syllable and not a letter, their writing system is called a *syllabary*, rather than an *alphabet*.

The clay tablets that Mesopotamian scribes wrote on were baked to preserve them. This process was so successful that many tablets survive even to this day. Most of what we know about Mesopotamian civilization we've learned through the translations of these cuneiform tablets, about 1,000 of which deal with medicine. In fact, from the ancient Sumerian city of Nippur comes the world's oldest known medical text—a cuneiform tablet that lists over a dozen prescriptions. The tablets also recorded epic tales of heroes and myths about gods and goddesses, bookkeeping, political documents, letters to and from kings, codes of law, accounts of battles, tribute lists, proverbs, treaties, hymns, and prophecies.

MESOPOTAMIAN RELIGION

The Mesopotamian world was filled with supernatural beings. The people believed in many gods, goddesses, devils, demons, and spirits. A major tenet of Mesopotamian religion held that humankind existed to serve the gods. The great temples in the Mesopotamian cities were enormous, complex structures each housing one particular god or goddess. Large staffs of priests and priestesses cared for the gods and performed numerous rituals, including feeding and clothing the image of the deity.

The people witnessed religious processions during festivals, but otherwise their religious practices did not involve the temples. Individuals had a personal god or goddess to whom they made offerings, prayers, and requests. The personal god interceded for the petitioner with the other gods and protected the person from the demons and evil spirits that inhabited the Mesopotamian world.

As is the case with many other ancient civilizations, health and religion went hand in hand in Mesopotamia. Demons, ghosts, or displeased deities were blamed for causing illnesses. A deity may be punishing the sick person because of offenses he or she committed or a demon may be carrying out the curse of the sick person's enemy. Pacifying the unhappy supernatural being or exorcizing the demon would bring relief.

Prayers and offerings were one way to appease the supernatural being causing the illness, if only the deity would listen. One poor sufferer wrote "My affliction increases, right I cannot find. I implored my god, but he did not turn his countenance; I prayed to my goddess, but she did not raise her head." Prayers to the gods for the punishment to stop often included confessions, such as, "My misdeeds are numerous, I have transgressed in every way," or "I have knowingly and unknowingly done wrong."

Divination—foretelling future events through signs in nature—represented another form of communication with the gods. Through divination, the diviner could predict the course of an illness and its outcome. Magic and sorcery of this type played an important role in Mesopotamian life, with spells and counter-spells for just about everything, especially for healing.

THE DOCTORS

There were several types of medical practitioners in ancient Mesopotamia, from magicians to priests to herbalists. Three types of healers, in particular, were held in high regard: the *asu,* the *ashipu,* and the *baru.* The *asu* were physicians and pharmacists, as well as members of the priesthood. The *ashipu* used magic and were also members of the clergy—exorcists, in a way. The *baru* were soothsayers whose main ability was the diagnosis of disease.

Rather than being rivals, though, these three types of medical practitioners sometimes worked together, perhaps with the understanding that illnesses take their toll on an individual both physically and spiritually. A sick man writes in an Assyrian letter, "Let him appoint one *ashipu* and one *asu*, and let them together perform their treatment on my behalf."

Sometimes the boundaries between the practitioners became blurred, since the *asu* occasionally used charms and the *ashipu* sometimes treated the sick with drugs. We even know of one man who was a deputy of the chief *asu*. Ten years later this man held the title of *ashipu*. Twenty-one years after that he was listed as an *asu* again.

AN EXORCIST'S INCANTATION AGAINST DEMONS

Thou art not to come near to my body,
Thou art not to go before me,
Thou art not to follow after me,
Where I stop, thou art not to stop,
Where I am thou art not to sit,
My house thou art not to enter,
My roof thou art not to haunt,
Thou art not to put thy foot in my foot's imprint,
Where I go thou art not to go,
Where I enter thou art not to enter.

THE ASHIPU

Scholars have translated the word *ashipu* as magician, sorcerer, exorcist-priest, and conjurer. These men (women were apparently not allowed to be *ashipu*) dealt with the world of demons and ghosts, of whom there were many in the Mesopotamian belief system. (Over 6,000 demons have been classified.) The *ashipu* had other duties besides healing, including ritually cleaning temples before religious ceremonies or working in the service of the king as an adviser. The *ashipu* performed all public acts of magic, overseeing the animals and other materials that were delivered to the palace for use in official rituals. *Ashipu* may also have visited the sick in their homes, counteracting omens or assisting in difficult times.

Ashipu presided over purification rituals designed to cleanse the patient who had contact with impure substances or people. One very elaborate royal ritual, known as House of Ablution, involved the Assyrian king and his *ashipu* going outside the city for several days, where the ritual would take place in a series of reed huts: "The king enters the fifth hut, while the exorcist recites the prayer formula 'Great Lord, Who in the Pure Heavens.' The king says the incantation: 'Shamash, Judge of Heaven and Earth.' You [the exorcist] set up a figurine of the Curse Demon, pierce its heart with a dagger made of tamarisk wood. He [the king] rinses his mouth with water and beer, spits it over the figurine. Then you bury it at the base of the wall."

This and other purification rituals involved water, oil, and other cleansing substances, such as potash, using rational techniques apparently for magical purposes.

Some tablets mention that an exorcist was the scribe, the owner, or both of medical texts. The *ashipu* had to be familiar with different texts: diagnostic omens, texts to quiet babies, magical texts about demons and ghosts, and information about plants, minerals, and animal substances and their uses.

The young student of magic started out as a scribe or apprentice magician, then became an *ashipu*, and ultimately might make chief exorcist. Sometimes demotions or dismissals occurred. In the city of Uruk, the temple of Anu had seven *ashipu*. The profession of magician passed from one generation to the next, and at this temple, *ashipu* came from only three clans.

The *ashipu* excelled at diagnosis. He interpreted the patient's symptoms and discovered the cause of the illness. He may have taken the patient's pulse, but most of the diagnosis relied on information from the *ashipu*'s handbook. The *ashipu* referred to the treatise of medical diagnoses and prognoses, comprising 3,000 entries on 40 tablets, divided into five sections—the largest collection of medical texts found so far. The title of this handbook comes from the opening line of the first chapter, "If the exorcist is going to the house of a patient," which was its title in antiquity. The form of each entry is done in the same manner. The first clause describes the patient's appearance or behavior and the second gives the prognosis. For example, "If [the patient] grinds his teeth and his hands and feet shake, it is the hand of the god Sin; he will die." The first two tablets in this collection, as the work's title implies, deal with what the *ashipu* might see on the way to the patient's house. "If the *ashipu* sees either a black dog or a black pig, that sick man will die. If he sees a white pig, that sick man will live."

The second section (12 tablets) lists the symptoms according to the body parts affected, starting with the skull and ending with the toes. The cause and the outcome are given. "If he is stricken by pain at the right side of his head: hand of Shamash—he will die."

The third section (10 tablets) lists the prognoses chronologically by the daily progress of the illness. The end of this section contains groups of symptoms indicating certain diseases. "If a man's body is yellow, his face is yellow, and his eyes are yellow, and the flesh is flabby, it is the yellow disease [jaundice]."

The fourth section consists of fragments of tablets mentioning treatments and describing certain syndromes. "If a man is stricken with a stroke of the face and his whole torso feels paralyzed, it is the work of the stroke; he will die."

The final section of six tablets seems to be about women's diseases, especially those stemming from pregnancy and malnutrition. The *ashipu's* prognoses were not always black and white—"he will live" or "he will die." Sometimes more detailed information is given—"he will live a long time but will not recover" or "he will die in three days."

Gods and demons did not always cause disease. Occasionally the patient's behavior brought about his misfortune—"he has had intercourse repeatedly with a married woman," or "he had sexual relations with his mother." The *ashipu* sometimes correlated the disease with a divinity; the goddess of love and voluptuousness, Ishtar, whose cult involved sacred prostitution, was often considered the cause of venereal diseases—a not entirely baseless assumption.

The *ashipu* relied on incantations to heal. Hundreds of these texts survive, going back to the middle of the third millennium BC. The practitioner directed these spells against demons, appealed to Shamash, the sun god, or sometimes just spoke nonsense words, like our "abracadabra." The *ashipu*, or sometimes the patient, repeated the incantation either three or seven times. The *ashipu* usually accompanied the incantation with some sort of action, the instructions for which followed the spell in the text. Often these actions involved setting up a brazier, preparing a censer, or making offerings to the divinity.

Often another type of practitioner contributed to a patient's case. The *baru*, or soothsayer, helped determine the cause of an illness, and how long it would last and sometimes determined if the patient should be treated or not. The *baru* did not form part of the temple priesthood but worked directly for the king as a scholar-in-residence or served local governments or the army. The *baru* also worked with other practitioners, such as dream interpreters, conjurers, and exorcists, on difficult cases as the following example from one of the ancient sources shows: "The *baru* through divination did not discern the situation. Through incense offering the dream interpreter did not explain my right . . . My omens have confounded the *baru*. The *ashipu* has not diagnosed the nature of my complaint, nor has the *baru* put a time limit on my illness."

Divination used a variety of signs from nature to predict the will of the gods or what would happen in the future, since the gods shaped the destinies of humankind. The word *baru* means examiner, and these men minutely examined a variety of natural occurrences and used these signs to foretell the future.

The omen collections come from the Akkadian period. These books provided the correct interpretation of signs, organized by topic. Thousands of these signs were collected into different series. One such series deals with the births of malformed humans and animals, and another discusses everyday events, such as the behavior of animals at the gates of a city or events occurring while building a house, performing agricultural tasks, or even washing oneself. Many of these omens predicted the health of an individual.

Another form of divination necessitated detailed examinations of nature; this type of foretelling used the internal organs of animals to acquire knowledge of the future. Unlike the omens mentioned above, the examination of animal organs belonged to a category of divination called "solicited omens," those that were actively sought out, rather than things that just happened to occur.

Extispicy, or gathering omens from the appearance of a sheep's entrails, was the most common form of soliciting omens. The sheep used for this purpose had to be carefully selected and magically purified. The *baru* then asked the gods to "write" their messages on the entrails.

Usually the liver of the animal contained the information that the *baru* sought after the dissection of the body. To help determine the omen from the appearance of the liver, the *baru* used clay models of livers that divided up the organ into rectangular areas with information written on each area locating important features. Archaeologists have discovered many such clay liver models throughout Mesopotamia. Thirty models came from a site called Mari, along with cuneiform tablets telling how to interpret the signs. The *baru*'s voluminous handbooks listed every possible deformity, mark, or discoloration of the liver, as well as the meaning of such abnormalities.

The interpretation of livers foretold a person's health, as in this example from the handbooks: "If a fleshy tumor is found at the bottom of the *na* (an unidentified part of the liver), the patient will get worse and he will die. If the liver passage falls to the right, the patient will live. If the gall bladder is long, the king will live long. If the *processus pyramidalis* is shaped normally, he who makes the sacrifice of the sheep will be in good health and live long."

Since divination from livers cost the inquirer the price of an animal, the *baru* also used cheaper forms of foretelling the future. One method involved the interpretation of the pattern oil made when poured on water: "When I let oil drop upon water, if the oil sinks and rises to the top again, it means misfortune for a sick man. If the oil forms a ring in the easterly direction, it means that a sick man will recover."

Another inexpensive way used the smoke issuing from a censer to make predictions. Astronomers or astrologers (they were considered the same thing) studied the heavens, noting celestial movements and weather phenomena, such as solstices, equinoxes, eclipses, thunder, rain, and hail. Predictions made from these observations related to the king, but sometimes they related to the health of important people.

Observatories throughout Mesopotamia sent regular reports to the king, which included a record of celestial happenings and interpretations of those events. Even very superstitious kings did not always listen to the omens. One diviner wrote to King Esarhaddon upbraiding him for his disbelief: "This is what the text says about that eclipse that occurred in the month of Nisan: 'If the planet Jupiter is present during an eclipse, it is good for the king because in his stead an important person at court will die,' but the king closed his ears—and see, a full month has not yet elapsed and the chief justice is dead."

THE ASU

In a hymn of self-praise, Gula, the Mesopotamian goddess of healing—often called "Great Physician"—describes herself in her role as an *asu*, surely reflecting human physicians' activities: "I am a physician, I can heal, I carry around all healing herbs, I drive away disease, I gird myself with the leather bag containing health-giving incantations. I carry around texts which bring recovery, I give cures to mankind. My pure dressing alleviates the wound, my soft bandage relieves the sick."

The *asu* were probably the closest to modern physicians. Their orientation toward remedies and drugs as therapy sounds more familiar to the modern ear than the magical cures of the *ashipu*. The *asu* relied on the correct herbal remedies for cures, along with incantations. From the description of Gula, we can assume that the *asu* probably carried a collection of herbs, incantations in a leather bag, and medical texts, as well as dressings and bandages. An ancient story describes a man who disguised himself as an *asu* by shaving his head and carrying a libation jar and a censer. If this was the disguise for an *asu*, then clearly, the *asu* used religious rituals as part of their healing practices and considered these spiritual measures as essential as the correct herbal prescription.

Little is known about the training of the *asu*. They were probably trained in cult centers—the vast temples found in various cities. The city of Isin was famous as a cult center of the goddess Gula, and a training center for physicians may have been located there. No formal apprenticeship programs existed, and much knowledge was surely passed on orally. However, some hierarchy existed in the profession because we know that the title *physician-in-chief* was used.

The medicine practiced by the *asu* almost certainly arose from a folk tradition of herbal healing. We read in a letter how one young physician gained knowledge of an herbal remedy: "The plants that your physician sent me are excellent. If there is a simmum illness [possibly malaria], that plant cures it immediately. I have just sent Shamshi-Addutukulti, the young physician, to you so that he can examine the plant. Send him back to me."

Obviously, the *asu* were willing to learn from their peers and share their knowledge. Most Mesopotamian medical treatments consisted of herbal remedies. The texts prescribe a variety of plant products, usually specifying the part to be used—leaves, flowers, seeds—prepared in a number of ways—crushed, cooked, dried, and so on. Pine, fir, and cedar resins were common ingredients. The *asu* mixed the plant matter with some type of liquid—water, beer, wine, or milk. Often some form of mineral was added as well. Healers used animal parts and even dung in their cures, too. Occasionally prescriptions warned the *asu* about the toxicity of certain ingredients. A letter from a physician to a high official shows the importance of obtaining exactly the right herb for a prescription. The doctor writes: "When I assigned a poultice for him, no *asu* herb was available. And my lord knows that if only a single herb is missing, it will not succeed. I asked the mayor to send word to a gardener . . . I gave her [a female patient] a potion for constipation to drink . . . but there is no *sarmadu* herb and drawn wine available. Let my lord send some . . . As to the herbs of which I spoke to my lord, let my lord not forget about them."

In about 500 BC, the *asu* Nabu-le'u wrote a document that gives us some insight into the medical practice of the *asu* and how they used their medical texts. The work is divided into three columns. The first column lists over 150 plants, indicating what part of the plant to use and stating any necessary precautions. The second column lists the diseases cured by these plants, and the third column gives details of how the medicine is to be taken—how often, the time of day, and if the patient should fast or not. Scholars call this type of medical text therapeutic because it gives prescriptions for treatment, unlike the diagnostic texts used by the *ashipu*, which give a diagnosis and prognosis, but no treatment. Sometimes therapeutic texts give a prognosis as well. The Mesopotamian

PRIVATE MATTERS— SAZIGA SPELLS

Private individuals also attempted to influence personal health matters. Saziga, or potency rituals, helped those suffering from impotence. Erotic incantations, recited sometimes by the man in question, sometimes by the woman, helped create a certain atmosphere. Along with incantations, people used herbal remedies, but unique to the saziga texts were prescriptions calling for items, sometimes sex organs, derived from sexually aroused or copulating birds or animals: "If a man loses his potency, you dry and crush a male bat that is ready to mate; you put it into water which has sat out on the roof; you give it to him to drink; that man will then recover potency."

The ashipu may have been involved in administering these prescriptions or it may have been a private matter. Other cures for impotence required the male and female genitals to be rubbed with special oils, occasionally with magnetic iron ore.

pharmacopoeia, reconstructed from the tablets of Assurbanipal's library, lists 250 vegetable substances and 150 minerals. Translations are not always certain, but material with known medicinal value may include aloe, anise, belladonna, cannabis, cardamom, castor oil, cinnamon, colocynth, coriander, garlic, henbane, licorice, mandragora, mint, and pomegranate. Other substances used in healing include fats and oils, animal parts, honey, and wax.

THE OLDEST MEDICAL TEXT

The earliest known record of medicine comes from Sumer. This document, written on a small clay tablet in about 2000 BC in the city of Nippur, reveals how physicians treated wounds. The "three healing gestures" used by doctors were: washing, making plasters, and bandaging. The tablet lists prescriptions using a number of raw materials. Twelve of these medicines were salves for external use, and eight were for plasters. One prescription for a plaster called for the physician to pound wine dregs, juniper, and prunes together. Beer would be added to this mixture to form the plaster, which would then be applied to the diseased part of the body.

AN ANCIENT PRESCRIPTION

If a man's tongue is swollen so that it fills his mouth, you dry tamarisk leaves, leaves of the adaru plant, leaves of the fox grape, and dog's tongue plant; you chop them up finely and sift; you knead them with juice of the kasu plant; you rub the top of his tongue with butter; you put the medication on his tongue, and he will get well.

Other medicines were liquids to be drunk, often dissolved in beer. One such prescription for internal use reads: "Crush to powder the seeds of the carpenter's herb, the gummy resin of the *markazi* plant, and thyme; dissolve in beer and give to the man to drink." Another prescription reads: "Pass through a sieve and then knead together: turtle shell, *naga-si* plant, salt, and mustard. Then wash the diseased part with beer of good quality and hot water, and rub with the mixture. Then friction and rub again with oil, and put on a plaster of pounded pine." Note that the physician washed the problem area before applying the mixture.

This little tablet also provides us with evidence for rather elaborate chemical procedures performed at this time. Saltpeter (potassium nitrate), a transparent, white crystalline compound, is mentioned. The physician probably got his saltpeter, used to draw torn tissue together, by crystallizing waste products from the canals. Alkalies, obtained by reducing a plant to ashes, were used to make plant extracts. The raw materials were boiled with salt and alkali and the solution was filtered.

The most amazing quality of this 4,000-year-old medical tablet is that, unlike later texts, nowhere is magic, demons, or sorcery mentioned. Medicine seems to have existed independently of sorcery, even at this early date. In later periods, the *ashipu*, or sorcerers, appear to have superseded the *asu*, or physicians, since the *asu* are not mentioned in later tablets. Although this may reflect the triumph of magic over medicine, it's often difficult to know whether the lack of written evidence means the *asu* disappeared or whether they stopped writing things down; perhaps the *asu* stopped recording their "secrets" simply because they didn't want their competitors to get their hands on them.

A VAST VARIETY OF CONDITIONS

What sort of illnesses and conditions did these medical practitioners attempt to cure or treat? In the tablets we read of migraines, insomnia, anorexia, impotence, anxiety, speech impediments, respiratory problems, liver disease, gastric troubles, enteritis, colic, diarrhea, intestinal blockages, dysentery, gout, jaundice, tuberculosis, pneumonia, bronchitis, hemorrhoids, stroke, gynecologic problems (including birth control), venereal infection, and mental illness.

Although the Mesopotamians believed that most illness came from supernatural powers, healers ascribed some conditions to natural causes such as cold weather, dryness, dust, putrescence, and malnutrition. They also understood the concept of contagion. Letters from the early second millennium BC speak of trying to control the spread of contagious illness by moving whole villages to higher ground.

Eye diseases occurred frequently in ancient Mesopotamia. The medical texts mention them often. Xerophthalmia, an eye disease that causes blindness in children, may have been widespread. This disease results from a lack of vitamin A. Physicians also treated ear problems, such as earaches, ringing in the ears, and hearing loss with pomegranate juice.

Dental problems troubled many Mesopotamians. Healers treated dental problems with incantations and a mixture of beer, malt, and oil. One text gives instructions for driving a pin into the tooth. King Esarhaddon's physician recommended the following: "The burning of his [the king's] head, his hands, his feet wherewith he burns is because of his teeth. His teeth should be drawn, his residence should be sprinkled. He has been brought low. Now he will be well exceedingly." Connecting fever with the teeth makes sound medical sense because in certain conditions, a hidden place of infection may be the cause, and today's physicians look carefully at the teeth in such cases.

Healers treated gastrointestinal problems, such as passing blood, rectal stricture, constipation, and flatulence, with suppositories and enemas. They may also have understood that the gallbladder could be involved in jaundice. One

Assyrian tablet mentions thick or cloudy urine, a sign of gonorrhea. Incontinence and gonorrhea were treated by introducing medicine through a bronze tube, a catheter, into the urethra. Many people had skin problems and these were treated with vegetable oils and animal fat applied to the skin.

Mesopotamian society seems rather dangerous when looked at through their laws. The code of Hammurabi refers to rape, kidnapping, destroying the eye of another, breaking another's bone, knocking out a tooth, striking a cheek, manslaughter, and being gored by an ox. A man "sick with a blow on the cheek" would receive the following treatment: "Pound together fir-turpentine, pine-turpentine, tamarisk, daisy, flour of *Inninnu*. Strain; mix in milk and beer in a small copper pan; spread on skin, bind on him, and he shall recover."

Physicians treated hemorrhaging from the nose with dressings, although some *asu* did not understand the correct use of the dressing. A letter from the chief physician to King Esarhaddon laments that the dressings that he prescribed for a patient were applied incorrectly: "The Rab-Mugi reported to me: 'Yesterday . . . much blood ran.' That is because the dressings that I had prescribed are applied without knowledge. They are placed over the nostrils, so they only obstruct the breathing, but come off when there is hemorrhage. They should be placed within the nostril; then they will stop the breath and hold back the blood. If it is agreeable to the king, I will go tomorrow and give instructions."

War wounds and other sorts of injuries would, of course, require the services of healers. The king of Mari received a letter from a remote military outpost begging him to send a physician because "if a slingstone wounds a man, there is not a single physician."

Midwives, called *sabsutu*, and female relatives assisted women in childbirth. Women giving birth used a birth stool; archaeologists have discovered clay models of them. Physicians often treated women for complications after the birth.

Many medical prescriptions existed for helping infertile women conceive and for easing the pain of labor and birth. One text gives a prescription for causing spontaneous abortion; eight ingredients are to be mixed in wine and drunk on an empty stomach.

On the other hand, an Assyrian law called for the death of someone who willfully self-aborted. If a woman had a miscarriage caused by a blow, the guilty party had to pay ten shekels for the loss of the child. The crime was not, however, willful miscarriage or abortion; it was the denying a man the right to sire a child within the marriage bonds that was the crime. If the woman herself died, the person who struck the blow would be put to death.

MESOPOTAMIAN SURGERY

Physicians were not limited to spells, external treatments, and herbs. Surgery was an option in some cases. Unfortunately, the medical texts tell us very little about surgery. The clay tablets mention the "bronze knife" only four times. Perhaps the *asu* learned this skill through observation, rather than by reading about it. The *asu* probably used his lancet for simple procedures, such as lancing boils, bloodletting, and perhaps cataract surgery. Tantalizing fragments of text describe cutting into the chest and scraping the skull to remove an abscess under the scalp. Even in ancient times, major surgery cost quite a bit. Ten shekels of silver—a not uncommon price—would have paid a carpenter's wages for 450 days!

Some evidence for trephination exists. This procedure involved sawing a square or round hole in the patient's skull to drain fluids and relieve pressure on the brain. Although texts do not mention the practice, trephined skulls have been found; one dating from 5000 BC comes from Arpachiya, four miles north of Nineveh.

After surgery on a scalp, the physician practiced a form of postoperative care. The medical text directs him to: "Wash a fine linen in water, soak it in oil, and put it on the wound. Crush powder of acacia and ammonia salt, and put it on the wound; let the dressing stand for three days. When you remove it, wash a fine linen in water, soak it in oil, put it on the wound, and knot a bandage over it. Leave the dressing three more days. Thus continue the dressing until healing ensues."

THE HAPPY, HEALTHY LIFE

Adad-guppi, the mother of King Nabonidus of Babylon, wrote an account of the end of her life, illustrating what health and happiness meant to this Mesopotamian queen mother: "The moon god added many days and years of happiness to my life and kept me alive . . . 104 happy years . . . My eyesight was good to the end, my hearing excellent, my hands and feet were sound, my words well chosen, food and drink agreed with me, my health was fine, and my mind happy. I saw my great-great grandchildren, up to the fourth generation, in good health and thus had my fill of old age."

ANCIENT EGYPT

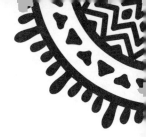

For many Americans, ancient Egypt means the pyramids, King Tut, and a host of questionable ideas derived from Hollywood. As one of the world's greatest civilizations, it often takes a backseat to Greece and Rome in classrooms. However, ancient Egypt was a civilization of enormous accomplishments in art, architecture, and especially the sciences—including medicine.

RELIGION AND HEALTH

The ancient Egyptians believed that each person was a product of different spiritual elements. Each person has a *ba* and a *ka*. *Ba* (often translated as "soul") vivifies the person but departs when the body dies; the *ba* is immortal. A person's *ka* is the element that fixes the person as an individual instance of their *ba*—a living, breathing animal. When the double spirits—the animal *ka* and the spiritual *ba*—live together in harmony, the individual lives a healthy and rewarding life.

Because both aspects of the person need nurturing, Egyptian medicine integrated physical and nonphysical aspects in its techniques. Prayer, medicine, and magic together played equally important roles in healing the whole person.

The Egyptians worshiped a great number of gods and goddesses. Many deities could assist those in need of medical care. People called upon specific benign deities to prevent or cure diseases and wild animal attacks. They directed incantations to disease-causing malign demons or deities, telling them to leave the body.

Some Egyptian temples were associated with healing and health care. One example is the temple of Hathor at Dendera where the buildings could be called infirmaries or sanatoria. Here the sick were cared for through baths, regimens, and special diets, as well as religious prayers. The temple of Thoueris is where priestesses acted as midwives for gynecologic and obstetric care.

Isis, one of the most important Egyptian divinities, had special powers to ward off evil and to undo the harm caused by malevolent forces. Isis's healing powers stem from the incredible feats she performed in Egyptian mythology, such as reconstructing her husband's chopped-up body and bringing him back to life. Isis showed great sympathy to even the lowliest members of society, and of all the numerous Egyptian divinities, people thought of her as the one most able to understand human suffering.

The son of Isis, Horus, also had a role in healing. He played a dual role as victim and savior. Those requesting medical help identified themselves with the injured Horus whose wound was healed. But Horus himself was also called upon to use his powers to heal. Some of his titles were "the good doctor" and "the savior."

Another deity people turned to for healing was Hathor, a sky goddess and the goddess of love, marriage, and motherhood. She was shown in art as a woman when relating to her role as sexual partner or as a cow when in her role as nurturing mother. Sometimes as a cow, she is portrayed with the Pharaoh suckling at her udder. Women giving birth prayed to her. In the Myth of Isis and Osiris, Hathor and the scorpion goddess Serqet attended Isis at the birth of Horus and helped nourish and protect him. Serqet also helped at the birth of kings and gods and protected embalmed bodies; she was a goddess of fertility and the afterlife.

The Egyptians tried to neutralize dangerous forces, such as poisonous scorpions, with kindness. If the goddess who controlled poison was treated well and given a great deal of respect, she could be convinced to use her power against scorpion bites. Some healers held the title "one who has power over the scorpion goddess." They tried to prevent and cure all sorts of stings and bites by persuading gods such as Serqet. The lioness goddess, Sekhmet, represented the forces of war and destruction, bringing misfortune, often in the form of infectious diseases. The Slaughterers of Sekhmet, dangerous demon messengers, brought flood, famine, and disease. Priests of Sekhmet, who specialized in medicine, tried to please this fearsome goddess with elaborate rituals to ward off plagues and pestilence.

The goddess Thoueris helped women in childbirth. She had the head of a hippopotamus, the arms and legs of a lion, a crocodile's tail, pendulous human breasts, and a prominent (pregnant) belly. Amulets often contained her image. Thoueris's appearance illustrates how the Egyptians combined all the dangerous and protective powers of a divinity in one image.

Thoth, the god of scribes, played a central role in Egyptian medicine and magic. He had special abilities in writing and reciting and was often called upon in healing incantations. In art, he appears as a baboon or an ibis (a long-legged, heron-like bird). In addition to the time that he restored Horus's eye, he is in the position of healer elsewhere in mythology: When a scorpion stung Horus, Isis made the sun stand still and caused such a disruption to the universe that Thoth went to help this mother in distress. He cured Horus with a spell. Of all the divinities, only Thoth, Isis, and Horus are called *swnw*, or doctor.

THE HEALERS: SWNW, PRIESTS, AND MAGICIANS

The word *swnw* (probably pronounced SUNU or SINU) means "doctor" or "physician" in ancient Egyptian. The *swnw* did not attend medical schools but trained with family members or as apprentices to masters. Their textbooks were the medical papyri. Some doctors may have owned their own texts, but since they were expensive, most probably consulted rolls in the House of Life. This institution, which was attached to various temples, served as a repository of papyri on a variety of subjects, including medical texts and works on purification, rituals, astronomy, and interpretation of dreams. Scribes read, copied, and perhaps composed the books kept there. The House of Life served as a library, scriptorium, and university. Physicians in training learned the art of the scribe in the House of Life, enabling them to read the medical texts kept there.

Physicians had a hierarchy with titles such as *administrator, overseer, inspector,* or *chief of doctors.* Royalty had personal physicians; during the Old Kingdom, almost half the doctors and dentists in Egypt were connected to the palace. Peseshet, a female doctor from the Old Kingdom, held the title of "female overseer of the female doctors." The only other known female physician was Tawe, from the Ptolemaic Period (332–30 BC).

We know little about individual doctors, how they practiced, or what they charged. The medical papyri tell us that the *swnw* examined his or her patient by feeling the abdomen or wound, as appropriate to the problem. The most important means of evaluation came from taking the pulses of the wrist, foot, stomach, groin, head, and neck. According to one papyrus, doctors examining wounds would pronounce one of three prognoses: An ailment which I will treat; an ailment with which I will contend; an ailment not to be treated.

Hery-shef-nakht, a physician from the Middle Kingdom, exemplifies how medicine, religion, and magic all formed an integral part of healing. He held the titles of chief of the king's physicians, priest of Sekhmet, and overseer of magicians. His duties included reading the papyrus rolls daily and examining and healing the sick.

The priests of the goddess Sekhmet played a role parallel, but possibly slightly inferior, to the *swnw*. Sekhmet, whose name means "power," symbolized might and terror. She brought pestilence and famine.

The need to appease Sekhmet gave her and her priests an important role in healing. The priests of Sekhmet may also have been veterinarians. *Swnw* and the Sekhmet priests did not compete against each other. In fact, some priests of Sekhmet also held medical titles, such as *Wenen-Nefer*, priest of Sekhmet, and medical inspector.

The priests of the scorpion goddess, Serqet, had a special role in treating the bites and stings of poisonous reptiles and insects. The Brooklyn Papyrus states that the ability to "drive out the poison of all snakes, all scorpions, all tarantulas, and all serpents . . . and to drive away all snakes and to seal their mouths . . . is in the hand of the priests of Serqet." The priests of Serqet accompanied mining expeditions into the Sinai because the danger of scorpion bites was so great in that region.

According to some sources, Egyptian physicians were masters of specialization. Not unlike today, Egyptian doctors specialized in fields such as ophthalmology, gastroenterology, proctology, and dentistry. They apparently had many doctors who would treat only one type of illness. Writing in about 440 BC, Herodotus, the Greek historian, notes: "Medicine is thereby divided among [the Egyptians] so that each doctor knows but one disease and none of the others. All [Egypt] is stuffed with physicians: Some appoint [themselves as experts] on eyes, others do the head, others teeth, others matters having to do with the belly, others specialize in hidden diseases." Although it is difficult to know whether Herodotus was exaggerating, clearly the Egyptians did make some distinctions among their medical experts.

KNOWLEDGE OF THE BODY AND DISEASE

Unlike modern medical practice, which relies heavily on postmortem studies for much of its anatomic knowledge, healers in ancient Egypt probably did not gain an understanding of anatomy from mummification. The Egyptians considered embalmers outcasts and objects of contempt because they came into contact with corpses and the causes of death. Although embalmers had some knowledge of anatomy, they probably had little contact with physicians and little opportunity to share their knowledge.

Instead, healers would have learned about anatomy from the slaughter of animals and from veterinary medicine, such as the highly prized cattle, which were treated by healers called "one who knows the bulls" and by the priests of Sekhmet. Medical practitioners would also have gained anatomic knowledge from the treatment of battle wounds and accidents that occurred during mining, quarrying, and building.

WEKHEDU IN THE METU

The ancient Egyptians had no knowledge of the circulatory system, but instead had a theory about *metu*, usually translated as "vessels" or "tubes." The metu included blood vessels, arteries, ducts, nerves, tendons, and muscles. These tubes ran between the heart and the anus and then went to various parts of the body carrying blood, air, mucus, urine, semen, water, and feces, as well as disease-bearing entities and good and evil spirits.

Disease arose when *wekhedu* traveled through the *metu*. Scholars have had a very difficult time translating *wekhedu*, but some suggestions for its meaning are "pain matter" or "morbid principle." The Egyptian theory of disease was based on the observation that after death, decay began in the bowels and then spread to the rest of the body. In the living, decay occurred in the bowels, therefore this internal decay could spread through the *metu*, causing disease. *Wekhedu* could develop in the body or enter from the outside. Once inside, it could stick to the fecal matter or pus and spread, causing dental problems, stomach cramps, eye infections, fevers, mental illness, and so on.

Because the Egyptians connected the cause of disease with food and digestion, the papyri stress moderation in eating and drinking; overindulgence caused internal illness. Herodotus, who visited Egypt, noted: "For three consecutive days in every month they purged themselves, pursuing after health by means of emetics and drenches; for they think it is from the food they eat that all sicknesses come to men."

The care of the anus—where *wekhedu* was known to develop—and proper elimination to get rid of *wekhedu* formed the basis of ancient Egyptian health maintenance. Most medical papyri discuss the anus, and a large number of prescriptions involved purges. Specialized physicians called "Shepherds of the Anus" gave enemas to ensure that *wekhedu* did not build up in the body.

Medical conditions were attributed to other causes, too. Some diseases were known to be caused by dietary or intestinal imbalances. Parasites, specifically worms, were another well-recognized agent of disease. But there were less tangible factors as well. Ethical or moral lapses could lead to divine punishment in the form of sickness. Magical forces brought about by the devices of enemies were another possible basis. It was also believed that in some cases change in climate could cause disease—a reasonable conclusion that we might attribute to the unfamiliarity of an individual's immune system with the local infectious agents.

DEALING WITH DISEASE

Parasites trouble Egyptians, even today. Schistosomiasis is a disease caused by worms that live in freshwater snails found on riverbanks. It causes urine in the blood, anemia, fatigue, loss of appetite, swelling of the scrotum, and can lead to bladder cancer. Schistosomiasis of the rectum, a painful condition, may explain the many remedies for "cooling and refreshing the anus." Many tomb paintings show men with umbilical hernias, scrotal swelling, and enlarged breasts—all symptoms of schistosomiasis. These conditions appeared mainly in men whose work brought them into frequent contact with river water—fishermen, boatmen, and papyrus gatherers. Egyptians may have tried to prevent schistosomiasis by avoiding contact with the river and by wearing penile sheaths, mistakenly assuming that infection occurred through the opening in the penis. Calcified eggs of the *Schistosoma* worm have been found in many mummies, including the unembalmed desiccated mummy of the weaver Nakht, from the New Kingdom. Poor Nakht was also infected with tapeworms and *Trichinella*, both caused by eating undercooked meat.

TREATMENT FOR PARASITES

Doctors prescribed many remedies for intestinal parasitic worms.

Herbal Substances	Mineral Substances	Animal Substances	Vehicles
• acacia leaves	• desert oil	• goose fat	• beer
• barley	• malachite	• honey	• milk
• bread	• natron	• ox fat	• wine
• carob	• red ochre	• white oil	
• dates	• salt		
• juniper berries			
• pine oil			
• sedge			
• sycamore figs			
• roots of pomegranate			
• wormwood/absinthe			

Hydatid disease, caused by eating food infested with the dog tapeworm, was also a problem. The disease causes cysts to develop in the organs, including the brain. These cysts have been found in mummies. Guinea-worm infestations occur when someone swallows water containing infected cyclops, a tiny crustacean. The worms can grow to as long as three feet. They perforate the skin of the ankle, forming an ulcer. The Egyptians tried to wind the worm slowly around a stick and out of the body when it showed itself. This could be dangerous if the worm broke. A mummy found with a calcified guinea-worm had had both legs amputated, perhaps because of a failed attempt at worm removal.

Some experts speculate that this treatment of winding the guinea-worm around a small stick may be the origin of the passage from the Bible in which the Israelites are plagued by serpents during their exodus from Egypt (Numbers 21:6–9). The Lord tells Moses to set a serpent upon a pole to cure the people. Perhaps this is a reference to guinea-worm infection and treatment. It is also possible that this ailment and treatment is the origin of the *caduceus*— the staff with a serpent coiled around it that has been the symbol of medicine for centuries. It is impossible to verify any of this speculation, however.

The Egyptians placed a great deal of emphasis on the idea of cleaning the bowels to prevent disease. *Swnw* must have been called in quite often to deal with constipation, since the medical texts give many remedies for clearing the bowels. These often involved the use of dates, figs, wormwood, coriander, cumin, juniper, malachite, and other herbs and minerals, combined with things such as honey, dew, wine, milk, or oil. One remedy calls for using the fruits or seeds of the castor-oil plant swallowed with beer. Linseed oil was used as a laxative; in fact, workers on the pyramids were issued a ration of the oil.

Ancient Egyptians' anuses apparently needed a lot of attention. One entire medical papyrus and 81 prescriptions refer only to the anus. Many remedies existed for cooling or refreshing the anus and for driving out heat. The prevalence of schistosomiasis would have created a great need for these cures. A suppository to cool the anus consisted of cinnamon, juniper berries, frankincense, ochre, cumin, honey, myrrh, and three other ingredients that are, unfortunately, as yet untranslatable.

The ancient Egyptians suffered greatly from dental problems. Many mummies show signs of periodontal disease, caused by stress applied to the teeth while chewing and by dental attrition—the wearing down of the teeth. Periodontal disease causes the teeth to loosen and fall out. Most ancient people had dental attrition, but the Egyptians seemed to suffer from it more than others, probably because the sandy soil contributed to a great deal of sand and grit in their food. Attrition wore down the teeth, exposing the dental pulp, which became infected, leading to abscesses and cysts.

Dentists, called *ibhy*, could also be *swnw*. They used various remedies to make firm or strengthen teeth loosened by periodontal disease. Some of these remedies involved the scraping of a millstone (a form of sympathetic magic) and the use of malachite or honey. A mixture of plants, carob, and honey was applied to ulcers of the teeth. Another remedy was cumin, incense, and carob applied as a powder.

Sand caused other problems for the Egyptians besides dental attrition. Sand pneumoconiosis—a noninfectious lung disease—occurs when people inhale blown sand. This condition still troubles those living in the Sahara and Negev deserts today. In ancient Egypt, everyone would have been exposed to the blowing desert sand; quarry workers and stone carvers were at greater risk.

Egyptian physicians were famous for their skill in treating eye problems, and several of them bore the title "doctor of the eyes." Many eye diseases were prevalent along the Nile. Leukoma, cataract, conjunctivitis, and trachoma (still known as the Egyptian eye disease) troubled people. And at least eight more eye diseases mentioned in the medical papyri have not yet been translated.

Eye treatments consisted of medication applied externally to the eye. Although other cultures seem to have experimented with cataract surgery, eye surgery did not exist in ancient Egypt. Remedies for blindness and poor eyesight included water from a pig's eye, pig bile, eye paint, honey, and fragments from an earthenware jar. One cure—eating liver—may have helped in cases of night blindness or xerophthalmia caused by a lack of vitamin A. Medicines for trachoma, a roughening of the eye, included bile of tortoise, laudanum, acacia leaves, carob, ground-up granite, eye paint, ochre, and natron. Eyelashes growing into the eye called for incense, lizard blood, and bat blood.

MEDICINES

Not only were the eye doctors of Egypt famous for their skill, but neighboring countries held all Egyptian physicians in high regard for their ability to prepare medicines. Ramesses II was asked to send a doctor to the Hittite court to prepare herbs for the king. In Homer's *Odyssey*, the famed Helen of Troy received a drug from the daughter of an Egyptian saying: "For in that land the fruitful earth bears drugs in plenty, some good and some dangerous; and there every man is a physician and acquainted with such lore beyond all mankind."

Prescriptions often indicate grinding, cooking, mashing, or straining the ingredients, which many times then "spend the night" in a vehicle such as water, alcohol, or oil. Often the active ingredient in the drug was an alkaloid extracted by soaking in alcohol in much the same way as a tincture. A typical Egyptian prescription follows (the fractions indicate relative proportions): "You shall then prepare for him to drink: figs, 1/8; milk, 1/16; notched sycamore figs, 1/8; which have spent the night in sweet beer, 1/10. Strain and drink much." Doctors sometimes gave patients a container of medicine with the prescription and instructions molded into the clay like a prescription label.

Incantations reinforced the effect of a remedy. This one was meant to be read when drinking the prescription: "The remedy comes, and there comes that which drives evil things from this my heart and these my limbs. Strong is magic in combination with a medicine and vice versa." The author of this spell had great faith in it. He notes that it's "Really excellent; it's worked a million times."

Medicines were also given rectally, vaginally, topically, and by inhalation and fumigation. Suppositories and enemas introduced drugs into the rectum. The gynecologic texts recommend cures and contraceptives for placement in the vagina. Physicians treated wounds with raw meat and then oil and honey. Diseases of the skin, hair, eyes, ears, and anus called for local applications of medicines, which were often bandaged in place.

Patients inhaled medicinal steam by means of a double pot. A liquid herbal remedy was poured over a heated stone placed in the bottom of a pot. Another pot was placed on top as a lid. A hole pierced in the bottom of the top pot allowed the patient to breath in the steam through a straw. Another treatment, fumigation, involved burning certain remedies and directing the smoke to the eyes, vagina, or any other affected areas.

MEDICINAL HERBS

The Egyptians probably had physic, or herb, gardens connected with temples. However, some herbs were gathered wild. The Ebers Papyrus gives us a glimpse into the gathering of a wild herb: "An herb—*senutet* is its name—growing on its belly like the kadet plant. It produces a flower like the lotus. If one finds its leaves looking like white wood, then one should fetch it and rub it on the pelvis." The Egyptians also imported plant products needed for medicine. Frankincense and myrrh came from Somalia. Pomegranate, olive, and fig trees came from elsewhere in the Near East or the Mediterranean.

MEDICINAL MINERALS

Many of the healers' drugs contained mineral products. Natron, an essential ingredient in mummification, drew out fluid and reduced swelling. The physician applied it externally and then placed a bandage over it. Salt occurred frequently in prescriptions and was used orally, in enemas and suppositories, and as an application to the eyes, ears, and skin.

Swnw often treated eye diseases with green eye paint, made of finely powdered malachite, mined in the Sinai. The traces of copper found in malachite would have inhibited the growth of bacteria. Healers also treated eye problems with lapis lazuli, a rare and valuable commodity, which the Egyptians imported from Afghanistan. Medicines contained other minerals, such as alabaster, alum, galena, clay, copper, granite, gypsum, hematite, Nile mud, ochre, and red lead.

ANIMAL PRODUCTS

Egyptian prescriptions contained a wide variety of animal products. Hundreds of remedies called for honey, which was used internally and topically. An ointment made with honey probably helped wounds because of honey's antibacterial and antifungal properties. It could also reduce swelling because its high concentration of sugar would draw out fluid.

Many prescriptions contained milk, usually as a vehicle rather than as an active ingredient. However, sometimes a specific type of milk was called for, such as the milk of an ass or human milk from a woman who had recently borne a son. In mythology, Isis brought her son Horus back to life by treating his burns with her own milk; therefore, people believed that the milk of a woman who had recently borne a son could transmit special healing powers.

Some drugs contained excrement from a variety of species, including cats, asses, birds, lizards, crocodiles, flies, and humans. Some treatments for eye problems called for the application of the excrement of a lizard, crocodile, pelican, or human. Rarely, fly and bird excrement was taken internally.

Blood from 21 species formed part of many external medicines. Human urine was an ingredient in enemas and was placed in the eyes. Cat placenta was part of a mixture to prevent hair from turning gray. A mouse cooked in oil also helped with this problem. Healers used goat bile to treat human bites and fish bile to strengthen eyesight. Physicians applied fresh meat to a wound on the first day. Greasy ointments often included animal fats. A rather surprising remedy for baldness required fat from a lion, hippo, crocodile, cat, snake, and ibex. Considering how exotic these creatures are, this treatment must have been very expensive. Ox liver, ass testicles, bird heart, and a variety of brains also played a role in drug preparation.

MEDICAL PROCEDURES

The papyri frequently mention the "knife treatment," but Egyptian physicians performed only minor surgical procedures, usually involving swellings, tumors, or snakebites. They did not attempt major operations. No surgical instruments have been found, and the famous carved relief of surgical instruments from the temple of Kom Ombo probably shows Roman, not Egyptian, objects.

Egyptian priests performed circumcision on boys in late puberty, usually as an initiation into manhood. Egyptian doctors rarely performed trephination— cutting an opening in the skull—but three examples of trephined skulls have been found. The trephined skull of a princess had well-healed edges, proving that she survived the operation.

Swnw normally treated a wound, such as a crocodile bite, by bandaging it with fresh meat immediately. After that, the healer bound the wound with oil and honey. Doctors did not use stitches except for gaping wounds, and no mummies have been found with suturing, except for one stitched after death. Sometimes the edges of a gash were drawn together with a bandage, though.

Healers applied a variety of substances to burns, including mud, excrement, resin, dough, oil, carob, papyrus, honey, ochre, malachite, and copper flakes. One burn remedy from the Ebers Papyrus comes highly recommended: "Barley bread, oil, and salt, mixed into one. Bandage with it often to make him well immediately. A true thing, I have seen it happen often for me."

For dislocated joints and fractured bones, healers used their hands to put them back into place. Archaeologists have found two bodies with bone fractures that had splints padded with linen and held in place with bandages.

POISONS

The priests of Serqet consulted the Brooklyn Papyrus for remedies for snake-bite. The text gives some spells, but most of this papyrus lists conventional remedies similar to those in the other medical papyri. These remedies are grouped according to the species involved or by the patient's symptoms.

The treatment of snakebites involved the care of the bite, the use of drugs, and magical incantations. Sometimes the priest incised the bite "with the knife treatment" and then applied salt or natron, held on with a bandage; this would potentially draw fluid, including the poison, out of the wound.

Many of the remedies for curing or preventing snakebite involved onions. One papyrus reads: "As for the onion, it should be in the hand of the priest of Serqet, wherever he is. It is that which kills the venom of every snake, male or female. If one grinds it in water and one smears a man with it, the snake will not bite him. If one grinds it in beer and sprinkles it all over the house one day in the new year, no serpent . . . will penetrate therein." Apparently, not every snakebite was treatable. Prognoses consist of blunt phrases such as "he will live," "one can save him," or "death hastens very quickly."

HEALTH CARE FOR WOMEN AND CHILDREN

Swnw did not specialize in gynecology and did not help women during healthy births. However, the medical papyri do mention contraception, conception, difficult births, and breast-feeding. The Egyptians did not understand female reproductive anatomy and believed that the womb wandered in the body. This caused a number of symptoms possibly along the lines of premenstrual syndrome. It was believed that during the monthly cycle, the womb would travel around the abdomen in search of sperm. Therefore, one treatment for wandering womb was intercourse. Another remedy recommends that the patient drink tar from a ship mixed with the dregs of "excellent beer."

A woman who wanted to become pregnant would drink the milk of a woman who had borne a son. To determine if a woman would bear a child and the sex of that child, one method suggested she urinate daily on two different kinds of wheat kept in two separate bags. If they both sprouted, she would bear a child. If the regular wheat grew, it would be a boy; if the spelt grew, a girl. If neither grew, she would not bear a child.

The Ebers Papyrus lists some remedies to hasten a birth. To cause the uterus to contract, hemp ground in honey or celery ground in cow's milk was prescribed. To "release a child from the belly of a woman," plants, resins, onion, beer, salt, and even fly excrement were placed in the vagina. During childbirth, women squatted on a birthing stool or on two large bricks. A midwife helped ease the baby out, then cut the umbilical cord with an obsidian knife.

Mothers breast-fed their children for up to three years. The papyri suggest testing the milk before feeding the baby. Bad milk smelled fishy. To make sure the mother produced enough milk, someone should rub the woman's back with a special mixture or feed her sour barley bread. Women who wanted to avoid pregnancy placed a variety of remedies in the vagina. To "allow women to cease conceiving for one, two, or three years," lint was moistened with acacia, carob, and dates ground with honey. Crocodile excrement features in some contraception remedies; the odor alone may have been enough to do the trick.

Infant mortality rates were high. Parents relied on charms and spells to protect children from spirits. People made amulets to protect babies by saying spells over beads and a seal with the image of a hand and a crocodile. The hand and crocodile would drive away evil that threatened the baby. The beads and seal, strung on a linen thread, were hung around the baby's neck.

THE HEALTHY PERSPECTIVE

In general, the ancient world did not have any illusions about their worldly lot. Few could expect to live past 40. One of the few to reach old age found much to complain about:

Age is here, old age arrived,
Feebleness came, weakness grows,
Childlike, one sleeps all day.
Eyes are dim, ears deaf,
Strength is waning through weariness,
The mouth silenced, speaks not,
The heart, void, recalls not the past,
The bones ache throughout.
Good has become evil, all taste is gone,
What age does to people is evil in everything.

Perhaps because life was so short, Egyptians held elaborate views of the afterlife and felt that in this life one should enjoy oneself. The most popular song in ancient Egypt reminded people to take advantage of every moment:

Spend a happy day.
Rejoice in the sweetest perfumes.
Adorn the neck and arms of your wife
with lotus flowers
And keep your loved one seated always at your side.
Call no halt to music and the dance,
But bid all care begone.
Spare a thought for nothing but pleasure,
For soon your turn will come to journey to the land of silence.

GREECE AND ROME

Greece and Rome dominate Western ancient history. Western art, literature, architecture, politics, and science all have their roots in these two great civilizations. Their influential legacy includes many of the basics of modern conventional, or allopathic, medicine but also some aspects of therapies now considered alternative. Prescribing plants as drugs, the extensive use of teaching texts, and even the modern conception of the physician as a scientist who trains by internship can be attributed to antiquity. Hippocrates, a Greek physician, is to this day heralded as "The Father of Medicine."

Of course, much of our modern reverence for this period comes from the fact that we have access to so much information about it compared with other civilizations. In classical times, knowledge was routinely recorded in written form and many ancient Greek and Latin texts were preserved through the Middle Ages in monasteries and, later, in universities. Textbooks, treatises, social histories, and even drug catalogs give us a pretty clear picture of medicine in ancient Greece and Rome.

GREECE

The earliest Greek references to the practice of medicine can be found in the works of Homer. Homer wrote in the eighth century BC about events that probably took place centuries earlier. Therefore, it is difficult to determine how many of the practices he mentions were in use at the time he was writing about or at the time he was actually writing. Practices probably did not change that significantly during that time, and certainly there is a heavy dose of myth that accompanies the accounts, so the distinction is not crucial.

Homer's works mention physicians who were considered professional public servants worthy of honor. In the *Iliad*, Asklepios could not leave his medical practice to participate in the Trojan War, so he sent his sons. The Mycenaean Greek warriors at Troy considered these physicians more valuable as healers than as fighters: "For a physician is a man worth more than many other men, both to cut out arrows and to spread gentle salves."

One son "sucked out the blood and skillfully applied gentle salves which once upon a time kindly Chiron gave to his father." Chiron was a centaur who was famous for his wisdom and knowledge of the medical arts and taught many heroes, including Asklepios.

The binding of wounds is mentioned twice in Homer. In fact, 147 wounds occur in the *Iliad*, and many are described with great precision, showing a rudimentary understanding of the anatomy of bones, muscles, and joints. When Odysseus received a wound, it was bound up, and a charm was recited.

Homer also mentions drugs coming from Egypt. Homer's "Egyptian drug" for wounds was probably opium; although opium does not itself come from Egypt, knowledge of the drug may have. Both the Minoans and Mycenaeans had extensive trade contact with Egypt and probably obtained medicines from the world-renowned physicians there.

GREEK RELIGION

As with almost all other cultures, religious beliefs played an important part in the early Greek concept of healing. Festivals honoring the gods included processions, dancing, hymns, and sometimes athletic, musical, or dramatic competitions. The gods directed human affairs, so keeping them happy with offerings was of the utmost importance.

By the fourth century BC, private religion centered around a new religious form: the mystery cults. These focused on a single god, and their membership was restricted to a few by invitation. The mystery cults taught that its worshipers would receive a form of immortality if they lived according to a code of ethical and religious behavior. The Eleusinian Mysteries was a cult that involved the worship of Demeter. Celebrating at the time of the autumn sowing, initiates took part in processions with torches, purification in the sea, fasting, and drinking barley water mixed with pennyroyal, a type of mint. The rituals culminated in some sort of revelation. Initiation in this cult would ensure happiness in the afterlife.

The worship of Orpheus was also a private religion. Orphism held that the body was evil and the soul divine. Initiates would also be guaranteed happiness in the afterlife. Followers of Orphism did not kill or eat animals.

The cult of Asklepios also formed a part of private religion, providing a close, personal relationship with the divine, not found in the state religion. Asklepios, as we'll see, was an important figure in Greek Medicine.

ASKLEPIOS, THE HEALER

The identity of Greece's greatest healer is murky. What is certain is that he had a significant influence over the practice of Greek medicine. His fabled techniques seem to be a mixture of incantations and pragmatic remedies—sometimes employing drugs and salves and sometimes invoking mystical powers. But his influence does not stop with knowledge of his renowned techniques.

Although a mortal in the *Iliad*, in later Greek mythology Asklepios (also spelled Aesculapius) was half divine—the son of Apollo, the god of healing, and Coronis. Chiron, the centaur, raised Asklepios and taught him the healing arts. Pindar, an early fifth century BC Greek poet, described Asklepios's career as a physician: "All those who came to him with ulcerous sores, with limbs wounded by grisly bronze or far-thrown stones, and with bodies ravaged by summer fever or wintry cold, each one he delivered from his special pain, treating some with soothing spells, some with healthful potions or spreading on their limbs ointments from far and near, or making them right again with the knife."

Asklepios's skill even enabled him to resurrect the dead, with the help of a plant that a serpent told him of. Zeus, enraged by the way Asklepios upset the natural order, struck him with a thunderbolt and killed him. After his death, Asklepios became a minor divinity, the worship of whom could bring health and prevent disease.

His family also had roles in healing. With his wife Epione, Asklepios had the two sons who took part in the Trojan War as healers, and two daughters who also had healing roles—Panacea and especially Hygieia, the personification of health.

ASKLEPIAN SANCTUARIES

This powerful reputation as a healer made Asklepios the object of popular worship. The Greeks built many cult centers to Asklepios where the sick could seek cures. Some of the most famous of the Asklepian sanctuaries were at Epidauros, on the Greek mainland; Cos, an island off Asia Minor; and Pergamum, in Asia Minor. These centers were located outside or at the edge of cities, in areas considered particularly healthful. They contained temples, gymnasiums, theaters, inns, priests' quarters, and baths—much like modern spas or retreats. Those wanting to ward off illness, to seek a cure for a disease or disability, or to give thanks for health followed a standard procedure after arriving at an Asklepian sanctuary.

First, the worshiper bathed in the sea, this outer cleansing symbolizing inner purity. The visitor next offered honey cakes on an altar and performed more ritual bathing at a water basin overseen by the priests. Those seeking a cure then entered the abaton, a sacred dormitory adjacent to the temple, where they would lie on pallets. Attendants put out the lights and encouraged silence and sleep. This sleep, known as incubation, formed the central part of the cure. During this sleep, Asklepios appeared to the worshiper in a dream or vision, carrying mortar, pestle, and a medicine chest. When the god healed the patient directly, he mixed potions, applied plasters, used the knife, or commanded the sacred serpent to lick the appropriate body part.

If Asklepios did not cure the patient himself, he gave instructions to the patient in a dream, to be performed when the patient awoke. When the god's recommendation was too difficult for the patient to understand, the priests would come in and interpret its meaning, prescribing drugs, a special diet, exercise, or baths. Those cured by Asklepios dedicated thank offerings to him in the form of sacrificed animals, cakes, money, wreaths, plates or cups of valuable metal, or models of the cured body part.

HIPPPOCRATES

Besides sacred healing in the Asklepian sanctuaries, Greek patients had access to secular physicians, too. These two healing systems, secular and sacred, coexisted without rivalry. By the Classical Period, the practice of medicine was revered, and doctors, although not deified like Asklepios, were prominent figures in society.

Hippocrates of Cos was a famous physician and teacher of medicine in the fifth century BC. He came to represent the ideal physician—devoted, kind, and skillful. He descended from a family of physicians that traced their roots back to the god Asklepios, and thus were called the "family of Asklepiads." As the family expanded, it became a guild of physicians. Two schools developed from this group; Hippocrates headed the school on the island of Cos.

THE HIPPOCRATIC CORPUS

Supposedly, Hippocrates wrote a large body of work, known as the Hippocratic Corpus, which includes the famous Hippocratic Oath. Scholars have argued since ancient times as to how many (if any) of these treatises were actually written by Hippocrates himself. Rather than the work of a single author, this group of medical writings is now regarded as the work of many authors and traditions, which had their origins in fifth and fourth century BC medical literature. When the librarians of Alexandria, Egypt, received any medical work, it appears that they classified it as having been authored by Hippocrates. It was the practice in ancient times to ascribe the works of an entire school to the founder, and students and disciples often wrote in the name of their master. Therefore, although Hippocrates himself may not have written any of this material, scholars still refer to the body of work as Hippocratic.

THE HUMORS

Social taboos prevented human dissection in fifth century Greece, limiting the knowledge of anatomy and physiology. To fill this gap in knowledge, the theory of the four humors was developed later in the Hellenistic period and attributed to Hippocrates along with the theory of pneuma. The four humors—blood, phlegm, yellow bile, and black bile—determined a person's constitution, temperament, and health. Pneuma (literally "air") allowed consciousness, thought, and perception.

An imbalance of the humors, caused by weather or diet, produced sickness. To regain health, seen as balance among the humors, physicians recommended purging, bloodletting, emetics, and dietary restrictions. The Hippocratic Corpus also contains material on herbal medicine, including the popular Greek purge made from black hellebore, parsnip, seseli, cumin, and anise.

DIAGNOSIS AND PROGNOSIS

Hippocratic medicine was concerned with prognosis, determining the likely course of an illness based on previous experience. Observation of the beginning and progress of the illness took into account the patient's appearance, noting especially breathing, sweating, excretion, and temperature. The physician looked for hollow, light-sensitive, or red eyes, cold ears, yellow skin color, and a tense face. He asked the patient about sleep, loose bowels, and appetite. Meno, a pupil of Aristotle, wrote that Hippocrates believed that gases emanating from undigested food rose through the body displacing health-giving breath. This theory resembles the ancient Egyptian idea of *wekhedu*. The Corpus also discusses diagnosis at length. Diseases are described, classified by symptoms, and explained. Along with the descriptions go lists of suitable foods, herbal remedies, and treatments for disease. As the following examples show, this work had elements of modern scientific method and practical applications for specific symptoms:

A consideration of the diet of the sick, as compared with that of men in health, would show that the diet of wild beasts and animals generally is not more harmful, as compared with that of men in health. Take a man sick of a disease which is neither severe and desperate nor yet altogether mild, but likely to be pronounced under wrong treatment, and suppose that he resolved to eat bread and meat, or any other food that is beneficial to men in health, not much of it, but far less than he could have taken had he been well . . . But as it is, if a man takes insufficient food, the mistake is as great as that of excess and harms the man just as much.

Here's another example:

Hydromel, drunk throughout the course of an acute disease, is less suited on the whole to the bilious, and to those with enlarged bellies, than to those who are not such. It causes less thirst than does sweet wine, for it softens the lungs, is mildly expectorant, and relieves a cough.

The Corpus also recognized the process of healing as a team endeavor:

Life is short and the Art (of medicine) long, the occasion urgent, experience deceptive, and decision difficult; yet not only must the physician be ready to do his duty but the patient, attendants, and circumstances must also cooperate if there is to be a cure.

THE HIPPOCRATIC OATH

Perhaps the most famous part of the Hippocratic Corpus is the Hippocratic Oath. Still used today as a declaration of a doctor's moral responsibility, it is one of the world's first statements of medical ethics:

I swear by Apollo, the Physician, and by Asklepios and Hygieia and Panaceia and all the gods and goddesses, making them my witnesses, that I will fulfill according to my ability and judgement this oath and this covenant:

To hold him who has taught me this art as equal to my parents and to live my life in partnership with him, and if he is in need of money to give him a share of mine, and to regard his offspring as equal to my brothers in male lineage and to teach them this art—if they desire to learn it—without fee and covenant; to give a share of precepts and oral instruction and all the other learning to my sons and to the sons of him who has instructed me and to pupils who have signed the covenant and have taken an oath according to the medical law, but to no one else.

I will apply dietetic measures for the benefit of the sick according to my ability and judgement; I will keep them from harm and injustice.

I will neither give a deadly drug to anybody if asked for it, nor will I make a suggestion to this effect. Similarly I will not give to a woman an abortive remedy. In purity and holiness I will guard my life and my art.

I will not use the knife, not even on sufferers from stone, but will withdraw in favor of such men as are engaged in this work.

Whatever houses I may visit, I will come for the benefit of the sick, remaining free of all intentional injustice, of all mischief, and in particular of sexual relations with both female and male persons, be they free or slaves.

What I may see or hear in the course of the treatment or even outside of the treatment in regard to the life of men, which on no account one must spread abroad, I will keep to myself holding such things shameful to be spoken about.

If I fulfill this oath and do not violate it, may it be granted to me to enjoy life and art, being honored with fame among all men for all time to come; if I transgress it and swear falsely, may the opposite of all this be my lot.

One aspect of ancient Greek medicine that distinguished it from other early forms of healing was its movement away from the understanding of illness as supernatural occurrence. Despite the Asklepian sanctuaries and various other private cults of healing, many of the great physicians of ancient Greece wrote about a rational, scientifically based view of biology and medicine.

The Hippocratic Corpus developed from observation and reasoning and contains no discussion of magic or superstition. Divinities did not cause disease, as in other medical belief systems. Diseases had their own individual natures and ran their course in a set time period. Humans were products of their environments, subject to the same physical laws as the rest of the world.

A Greek physician who studied at Alexandria, Soranus practiced his art in Rome in the second century AD. Although he wrote about 20 books, only 2, on fractures and on gynecology, have survived. His works offer rational and practical advice, sound therapy, and a denunciation of superstition. Soranus wanted to remove all superstition from medicine because he felt it was at best useless, and often involved unpleasant, painful, or dangerous treatments. However, he did recognize the value of harmless objects, such as amulets, saying: "One should not forbid their use; for even if the amulet has no direct effect, still through hope it will possibly make the patient more cheerful."

The ancient Greeks believed hysteria was caused by problems with the uterus (*hystera* is the Greek word for uterus or womb). Many Greek physicians treated this condition with unpleasant methods, such as anointing the nose and ears with burnt hair or squashed bedbugs or by blowing air into the uterus. In contrast, Soranus recommended such reasonable treatments as warm compresses and relaxing baths.

THE BOTANISTS, EARLY PHARMACISTS

The prescribing of drugs was a significant part of Greek medicine, but drugs in those days were mainly herbs and other plant products. Therefore, herbalists or botanists were the true pharmacists. Several great Greek botanists distinguished themselves, leaving behind a huge body of work on the classification and medicinal uses of various plants.

Theophrastes. Aristotle's pupil, colleague, and successor, Theophrastes was not technically a physician but a philosopher and, one might say, a pharmacist of sorts. He made the first systematic study of plants using observation and classification; his work is considered antiquity's highest achievement in botany. Theophrastes wrote about herbal medicine, detailing the plant parts used, the methods of collection, and the herb's effects on people and animals.

Diokles. Theophrastes was not the first Greek to write a medicinal herbal. The late fourth century BC physician Diokles holds that honor. Athenians called Diokles a "younger Hippocrates" and credited him with inventing a type of head bandage and an ingenious device for extracting barbed arrows from wounds called the "Spoon of Diokles." Only fragments of his works on animal anatomy, botany, physiology, and dietetics survive, but Theophrastes seems to have used Diokles's material as a source in his own writings.

Dioscorides. Pedanius Dioscorides was a Greek physician and botanist who lived during the first century AD. Dioscorides probably traveled extensively and discussed cures with a wide variety of people. He matched testimonies with scientific observation and scholarly research into the work of other pharmacy experts whose work is now largely lost.

He compiled his knowledge into a systematic, rational treatise on the medical property of 600 plants, 90 minerals, and 35 animal products, including the flesh of vipers. This work, produced in Greek, was translated into Latin, Arabic, and in 1665, into English; it is the most widely read botanical work ever written. Dioscorides's work greatly influenced Islamic, medieval, and renaissance botany and medicine.

LEARNING ABOUT ANATOMY

A crucial window of time for the study of anatomy opened up in Alexandria during the

THE HERBS OF THEOPHRASTES

The following entries are from Theophrastes's botanical writings (when he refers to "they," he is speaking of the various peoples of the empire from whom the recipes and uses were learned):

The root of cyclamen [part of the primrose family] is used for suppurating [discharging] boils; also as a pessary for women and, mixed with honey, for dressing wounds; the juice for purging of the head, for which purpose it is mixed with honey and poured in; it also conduces to drunkenness, if one is given a draught of wine in which [the root] has been steeped. They say also that the root is a good charm for inducing rapid delivery and as a love potion; when they have dug it up, they burn it, and then, having steeped the ashes in wine, make little balls like those made of wine-lees [dregs], which we use as soap.

The root of wild cucumber [squirting cucumber] is used for white leprosy and for mange in sheep, while the extracted juice makes the drug called "the driver." It is collected in autumn, for then it is best.

The leaves of germander pounded up in olive oil are used for fractures and wounds and for spreading sores; the fruit purges bile and is good also for the eyes; for ulcers in the eye, they pound up the leaf in olive oil before applying it. It has leaves like the oak, but its entire growth is only about a palm high; and it is sweet both to smell and taste.

Hellenistic period in the third century BC. Before then, Greek religion and custom forbade human dissection; by the second century AD the practice had ended.

Herophilus, the Anatomist.
Herophilus (fourth century BC), a Greek physician and medical scholar trained in Cos, went to Alexandria. There, dissection and even vivisection of condemned criminals was performed. He applied logic to direct observation and made important discoveries about the eye, liver, brain, and the reproductive, vascular, and nervous systems. He identified nerves but thought they were channels for pneuma (the word for "air" that also came to mean "thought")—a not altogether wrong assertion. Herophilus discovered that the brain was the location of intellect, believing it the center of the nervous system. He may have been the first to discover the fallopian tubes and ovaries. Herophilus did not simply study the body, though; he tried to use his anatomical knowledge, along with recommendations about diet and exercise, to restore and maintain health.

Erasistratus, Father of Physiology. A contemporary of Herophilus, Erasistratus (born ca. 304 BC) was a Greek physician trained at Athens and Cos. After emigrating to Alexandria, Erasistratus furthered the anatomic researches of Herophilus, advancing knowledge of the brain, heart, and nervous and vascular systems. His primary interest was physiology (the study of the workings of the body), particularly respiration and digestion.

THE WONDERS OF LETTUCE

The following are entries from Dioscorides's work De Materia Medica:

Cultivated lettuce; good for upper tract, a little cooling, sleep causing, softening to lower tract, increasing lactation. Boiled down it increases nutrition. Unwashed and eaten it is given for upper digestive troubles. Its seeds being drunk are good for [those who] continually dream and [the seeds help the patient] avert sexual intercourse; eaten too often they cause dim-sightedness. They are preserved in brine. The stalk growing up has something like the potency of the juice and sap of wild lettuce.

Wild lettuce is similar to the cultivated, larger stalk; leaves: whiter, thinner, more rough, and bitter to the taste. To some degree its properties are similar to those of opium poppy, thus some people mix its juice with opium. Whence its sap, 2 obols [1.14 grams] in weight with sour wine purges away watery humors through the digestive tract; it cleans away albugo [a white opacity of the cornea], misty eyes. It assists against the burning [of eyes] anointed on with woman's milk. Generally it is sleep inducing and anodyne. It expels the menses; [it is] given in a drink for scorpion and venomous spider bites. Drinking the seeds, similar to that of the cultivated kind, averts dreams and sexual intercourse. Its juice produces the same things [as cultivated lettuce] but with a weaker force. The sap [should be] extracted in an earth bowl, exposed to sunlight first . . . and stored.

Erasistratus also worked as a surgeon, opening the abdomen to treat the liver and using catheterization to treat slow, painful urination. Going against the teachings of the Hippocratic Corpus, Erasistratus was skeptical of bloodletting and the theory of the four humors.

GALEN: A PHILOSOPHER DOCTOR

Galen, the last great ancient thinker in the field of medicine, lived in the second century AD. A Greek from Pergamum in Asia Minor, he studied grammar, logic, and philosophy before beginning his medical studies at age 16 in Egypt. He returned to his hometown to take a post as doctor in a gladiator school. From there he moved to Rome where he became physician to the emperor Marcus Aurelius, began a large medical practice, lectured on anatomy, and vivisected and dissected animals, especially apes. Galen performed important work using dissection, proving that both arteries and veins carry blood—a landmark discovery in Greek medicine and medicine in general.

In addition to his contributions to anatomy and physiology, his works contain information on pharmaceuticals; the term *galenic* refers to his principles of using plant preparations. A galenical is a vegetable remedy or herbal simple. He also concocted a form of *theriac*, the famous panacea containing almost 70 ingredients in an opium base (see "Theriac—A Popular Panacea").

Galen wrote on many topics, including philosophy, anatomy, pathology, and therapy. He felt that philosophy and medicine should be integrated. He was a monotheist who felt that the study of anatomy was a way of praising God.

THERIAC—A POPULAR PANACEA

Galen did not invent it, but he produced this popular remedy for the Roman Emperor Marcus Aurelius. The name *theriac* comes from the Greek word for wild animal. Theriacs were originally antidotes to both human and animal bites, which the ancients thought to be poisonous. They were then used against poisons in general.

The Persian king Mithridates poisoned criminals to study the effects of antidotes; he compounded the most effective ones into a drug for his own use, which he named mithridatium, after himself. Andromachus, the Roman Emperor Nero's physician, took mithridatium, now called theriac, added chunks of viper flesh to the recipe, quintupled the amount of opium, and brought the total number of ingredients to 64. Galen applied theriac to bites and abscesses and wrote a whole book on the subject. Theriac was a popular panacea through the ages; it remained in the official French pharmacopoeia until 1884.

Galen's comprehensive system of medical philosophy came to be the embodiment of Greek and Roman medical knowledge; it dominated medicine for over a thousand years.

THE HEALTH CARE SYSTEM

Although some of their techniques were primitive, the ancient Greek system of health care evolved into one that, in many respects, looks like our modern Western one. Their education and training followed similar lines, and they even had private offices.

Originally medical knowledge was handed down through the family. Healing was generally a private matter, but medicine slowly developed from a skill to a trade. Physicians were eventually considered workers for the public good. They traveled from place to place with instruments, appliances, and drugs, examining patients.

Many physicians had apprentices bound by an agreement. The masters imparted their secrets to their apprentices directly. Then, special centers for the study of medicine began to appear in east Greece at Cos and Cnidus, at Cyrene and Alexandria in North Africa, and in Italy at Croton. These centers were free associations of physicians, teachers, students, and apprentices. Physicians received employment from rulers or cities as public physicians, or they set themselves up in private practice. Doctors examined and treated the sick in an *iatreion*, or physician's office, equipped with special lights, instruments, bandages, and drugs. They prepared the drugs themselves or with the help of a root cutter, who collected, dried, pulverized, and prepared roots and plants for use as remedies—the ancient equivalent of the pharmacist.

GREEK DRUGS

Greek physicians prescribed a wide variety of drugs, some effective and some actually harmful. They poured vinegar or wine into wounds and over dressings as a disinfectant. Physicians gave hellebore, a poisonous plant, to patients to induce vomiting and diarrhea.

Inflamed wounds were covered with a plaster made from mullein, raw clover leaves, boiled rock plant, and hulwort. Greek physicians and botanists ascribed different uses to hundreds of plants. For example, mustard had more than its share of medicinal duties. Hippocrates recommended white mustard seed taken internally or applied as a counter-irritating poultice made with vinegar. Dioscorides stated that mustard leaves are good for internal pain of long duration. Mustard juice mixed with honey and water was a good gargle for inflamed tonsils. Used as an ointment, mustard cured dandruff and cleared the complexion. Added to figs, it improved hearing, whereas mustard juice in honey helped the eyesight.

Minerals also had a place in Greek pharmaceuticals. Powdered alum, sodium carbonate, copper oxides, lead oxides, and lead sulfate dried and disinfected ulcers and wounds. Animal products occasionally played a role in drug preparation. Viper's flesh was one of the more popular animal ingredients. Snake meat pickled in oil, wine, salt, and dill was used to improve eyesight and nerves. Physicians recommended using drugs in a variety of ways. Patients took them internally, applied them externally as salves, ointments, and plasters, and sat over burning substances or vapor baths containing herbal remedies. Pessaries consisting of remedies wrapped in wool or linen were inserted vaginally, and enemas were used for purging.

THE HEALTHFUL REGIMEN

Although it seems remarkable how similar ancient Greek medical practices are to our own—or, more accurately, how much our practices are based on the Greek—one aspect of treatment they emphasized that is only now making a resurgence in modern medicine is lifestyle adjustments. Regimens—integrated courses of treatment involving diet, exercise, rest, and personal hygiene—were often part of Greek health practices. And prevention rather than treatment was often the aim of these regimens.

Ancient Greek healers believed the right foods and exercise, applied with attention to the seasons, winds, age, and home situation of the individual, could prevent illness. Humans, being composed of fire and water, had to keep these two elements in balance with a healthful regimen. Foods were considered to have actions congruent with elements, such as cooling, drying, heating, wind-producing, moistening, binding, and so on. For example, barley was considered cooling and drying, millet was dry and binding, fish were dry and light, wines were hot and dry, garlic was hot and laxative, and so on. While recovering from illness, patients were fed barley gruel, honey and water, honey and vinegar, and a variety of wines.

Different forms of exercise also helped keep the body in balance. Running heated and dissolved the flesh and digested the food; wrestling hardened the body. (You could pay a professional trainer to tell you the same today.) Walking, ball playing, sparring, and marching were all recommended. Hippocrates and Galen endorsed massage for toning the body. Strenuous rubbing hardened the body and gentle rubbing relaxed it.

MEDICAL PROCEDURES

Greek healers treated a variety of injuries and diseases. The Hippocratic Corpus mentions many war wounds: a man hit high in the abdomen with a powerful and dangerous arrow, someone wounded in the back with a javelin, a man wounded from behind by a broad lance, and so on. Industrial accidents also took their toll: A man who fell on an anchor was wounded in the belly, a loaded wagon passed over a man's chest and broke his ribs, and a cobbler stabbed his thigh with the awl. Often physicians prescribed enemas, purges, and emetics for such injuries. Even minor injuries could lead to death from tetanus or erysipelas—a spreading inflammation caused by bacteria, sometimes associated with gangrene.

Besides purges and emetics, physicians used fomentations (the application of heat), bleeding, cautery, draining of the lungs, and suturing to treat wounds. Skins, bladders, and bronze or pottery vessels held hot fomentations, recommended for pain in the side. Bleeding was achieved by venesection, leeches, or cupping. Greek physicians used bloodletting with cups so frequently that the bleeding cup became the symbol of the physician and was often depicted on doctors' tombstones. Bleeding was used to cure many ailments including eye disease, pneumonia, and lack of nourishment from food. Physicians used cauteries (heated irons) for many different procedures, such as destroying abnormal growths, curing or preventing dislocations, stopping hemorrhage, and draining pus from the lungs. The main purpose of cauterization was to drain by piercing a hole or to dry and tense particular parts of the body.

MIDWIVES

Although female physicians were not the norm, the profession of midwife was well respected. Greek midwives were expected to read and study medical texts. Herophilus, Soranus, and Galen all wrote treatises or practical manuals for midwives. Midwives performed much the same service as a doctor, having some knowledge of medical theory. Midwives also worked under the direction of male physicians, serving as intermediaries between doctor and patient.

In the words of Soranus: "The midwife must have the right mental, moral, and physical qualifications: She must be literate and study her work theoretically. She must have a keen understanding and a good memory; must enjoy her work and have a sense of honor; must have sound sense, a strong constitution, practical experience, and presence of mind; must not be easily alarmed, but must be sympathetic; that she should herself have given birth is not absolutely necessary. She should further be strong, steady, not given to talk, proof against bribery by those who desire criminal abortion, and free of superstition. She must have gentle hands."

Childbirth took place in the home of the pregnant woman. The midwife made sure that all necessary equipment was available. This included a birthing stool, oil for injection and lubrication, warm water for cleansing, warm fomentations to ease pain, sea sponges, pieces of wool, bandages for swaddling, a pillow to place the baby on, and things to smell, such as pennyroyal, apples, and quinces.

Midwives controlled the birth, although a physician might be present to oversee the proceedings. The midwife checked the progress of dilation. When enough space existed for the passage of the baby, the woman got up from her bed and sat on the birthing stool. The seat was crescent shaped; the sides were solid boards with handles that the woman grasped and pressed while straining. The front and back were open to allow access by the midwife and her assistant.

The Hippocratic Corpus mentions numerous methods of birth control and abortion. For example, to prevent pregnancy for one year, a woman should soak a piece of copper sulfate in water and drink the liquid. Copper is used today to make certain intrauterine devices (IUDs) because copper is a spermicide. The Corpus also advocated the Lacedaimonian leap—leaping with the heels to the buttocks, squatting, and sneezing violently to expel the man's seed.

Soranus had more to say on the subject. He recommended that when the man was about to ejaculate, the woman must hold her breath and draw away a little, so the seed would not be hurled too deeply into the uterus. She should get up immediately, squat, induce sneezing, wipe the vagina, and drink something cold. He also suggested smearing the orifice of the uterus with olive oil, honey, cedar resin, balsam tree juice, or white lead. He mentions vaginal suppositories and oral contraceptives containing botanical ingredients such as pomegranate peel, silphium (a now-extinct plant in the giant fennel family—the tree, not the herb), rue, and rocket. Many of the plants that Soranus recommended have been shown through modern testing to have an effect as a contraceptive or abortifacient. Women also used amulets and charms as contraceptives. For a woman who sought an abortion, Soranus recommended that she should take violent exercise, be jolted in a carriage, and should carry heavy things. Other means of inducing abortion were vigorous massage, the eating of spicy foods, using diuretics and clysters to purge the abdomen, and a variety of poultices and vaginal injections. When all else failed, protracted baths and heavy bloodletting were used.

ROME

So closely linked were the Greek and Roman cultures that it is often difficult for us to look back and distinguish exactly who gave us what. Even during the height of Roman power, most of the Mediterranean world they controlled used the Greek language, not Latin. Greek was the common language of the Mediterranean world. In fact, many of the aristocracy in Rome itself used Greek well into the first century AD. Some of the great Greek physicians named earlier—Dioscorides and Galen among them—lived under Roman rule and served, however distant, the Roman emperors.

Early Roman healing contained a strong religious element. People who were seeking protection and health would pray: "Father Mars, I entreat and beg you . . . to keep at bay, repulse, and take away disease, known and arcane . . . and to give health to me, my house, and my household." Prayers and offerings were also made for the health of cattle—supernatural veterinary medicine.

Healing sanctuaries existed throughout the lands conquered by Rome. Most centered on hot or cold mineral springs. Ponte di Nona, a healing sanctuary established in the late fourth century BC near Rome, contained a temple, a circular pool, a small hostel with baths, and an enclosed mineral spring. People seeking or giving thanks for healing dedicated many votive offerings there, such as terra-cotta hands and feet, heads, eyes, and sexual organs—images of what had been healed or what needed healing.

A popular healing sanctuary at a spring site in Umbria contained a temple to the god Clitumnus. The sanctuary also held small shrines, each with its own god; some of these had their own springs. Archaeologists have uncovered many votive tablets expressing the gratitude of the healed and of those to whom Clitumnus revealed the future.

AGRICULTURAL BEGINNINGS OF MEDICINE

The beginnings of Roman medicine come from agriculture. The *pater familias* administered cures to family, slaves, and farm animals. These cures consisted of incantations and animal, vegetable, and mineral remedies. Wool was believed to have numerous curative powers when combined with other ingredients, such as fat, rose oil, honey, sulfur, vinegar, and the herb rue. Cabbage also had many uses as a remedy. Even the urine of a person who had been living on cabbage was used; children who were washed with it would never be weak and puny.

Early Roman medicine involved treatment with simple remedies; issues of prognosis, diagnosis, and prevention were not addressed. The person who administered the cure needed no special training, and doctors played no part in this form of healing.

Eventually, the Romans began to adopt the methods and theories of the visiting Greeks. A Roman physician, like a Greek one, trained with a doctor father or served as an apprentice. Sometimes a teacher would take students with him while visiting patients or would give medical lessons in his shop, called a *taberna medica*. Some cities hired doctors to give medical instruction and to treat the needy for free. Most physicians would not have had access to books or drawings but could visit centers of medical studies to consult references. Like artisans, physicians formed guilds, which had their own offices and secretaries. These guilds met to discuss work-related affairs, to give advice and instruction, and to provide meals and burials for members.

A ROMAN RECIPE FOR TREATMENT OF ASTHMA AND POISON

- 1/2 hemixeston (about 1 pint) nut grass
- ripe juniper berries
- 12 minas (about 9 pounds) plum raisins
- 5 minas purified pine resin
- 5 minas sweet flag
- 1 mina camel's thorn
- 12 drachmas (1 1/2 ounces) myrrh
- 9 sextai (18 ounces) old wine
- 2 minas honey

Having removed the seeds from the raisins, pound and crush them with the wine and the myrrh, and having pounded and sifted the rest of the ingredients, combine them all to soak for one day; then, having boiled the honey until it has a glutinous consistency, mix it carefully with melted pine resin, and having carefully pounded together the rest of the ingredients, put up for storage in an earthen vessel.

PLINY AND CELSUS

Pliny the Elder (AD 23–79) wrote the *Natural History*, a compendium of scientific knowledge covering a number of topics. Of the 37 volumes, seven cover medical botany. Pliny discusses at length the medicinal qualities of many herbs, vegetables, and minerals. He had little faith in physicians and herb sellers, many of whom he felt were quacks. Echoing an anti-establishment opinion you're likely to hear from some quarters today, Pliny thought that: "if people sought remedies in the kitchen-garden, medicine would be quite cheap. But herbs are not familiar to most people because experience of them is confined to country folk, who live among the herbs; moreover, nobody wants to look for herbs when crowds of medical men are everywhere."

Aulus Cornelius Celsus wrote his encyclopedia on agriculture, medicine, military science, rhetoric, philosophy, and law during the reign of the Roman emperor Tiberius (AD 14–37). Celsus, a wealthy Roman landowner, summarized medical knowledge down to his own time, including the native Latin traditions and the theories of the Hellenistic medical schools. Pliny and Celsus provide us with a look at Roman health, healing, and the various cures and practices available during the first century AD.

PREVENTIVE MEDICINE

Romans excelled at public hygiene. Since the earliest times, swamps were drained to prevent disease. When building fortified towns, the Romans sought out sites, away from swamps. The Cloaca Maxima, the main sewer of Rome, drained waste into the Tiber River. Aqueducts ensured a clean water supply for the city. Public baths allowed all classes of society to maintain cleanliness.

In addition to public hygiene, the Romans also recognized the influence of lifestyle factors on health. Celsus recommended the preventive called "the regimen": regulating food, drink, exercise, bathing, and medicine. Celsus's regimen included moderation in food and drink. Dessert, for those who could take it, should consist of dates or apples. For exercise, Celsus favored walking, the strenuousness of which depended on the constitution of the individual.

Massage was also revered by the Romans. They used it for toning, fever recovery, and to relieve headaches and partial paralysis. The wealthy had personal physicians and assistants who massaged them at home. Others got massage treatments at public baths where trainers and doctors sold their services.

ROMAN DRUGS

A Roman doctor's office would have shelves and cupboards to hold medical instruments and herbs and drugs in jars, pots, and boxes. Equipment for drug preparation, such as mortar and pestle, balances, marble palettes for rolling pills, bottles, scoops, spoons, and spatulas would all be needed. Animal fats, wax, olive oil, wine, water, milk, and honey were used in drug preparation as well.

CELSUS ON EXERCISE

For the person who has been occupied during the day, whether in public or private matters, should designate some part of the day for the care of his body. His first concern in this regard should be exercise, which ought always to precede the eating of food. The exercise should be greater for him who has worked less and is considered well, and it should be lighter for him who is tired and who has thought less during the day . . . A healthy man, who is both strong and his own master, ought not to place himself under any arbitrary rules, nor should he have a need for a doctor . . . His sort of life should give him variety. He should sometimes be in the country, sometimes in the city, more often should he be on a farm. He should sail, hunt, rest from time to time, but more frequently exercise his body. While inactivity weakens the body, work makes it strong; the former gives an early old age, and the latter promotes an extended youth.

Besides the pharmacopoeias, which listed hundreds of plants and their uses, the Romans learned of medicinal plants from their allies. In a fortress in Germany, the lid of a pot with the words "Extract of the root of britannica" was found. Pliny tells us of camp where the soldiers suffered from scurvy, their teeth falling out and their knee joints failing. The Frisians, a tribe then loyal to the Romans, introduced them to the plant called britannica, which was good for the sinews and mouth diseases and relieved quinsy and snakebite. This plant has been identified as water dock (from the genus *Rumex*). Seeds of dock have been found in several Roman towns in Britain.

Eye diseases troubled many in the Roman Empire to the point where all recruits going into the Roman army had to take an eye test. Eye ointments and salves constituted a major part of ancient pharmacopoeias. Salves were often named for their inventor, such as the salve of Axius or salve of Philo. Some salves contained minerals—copper and zinc hydroxide, zinc carbonate, and mercuric sulfide—that would have been helpful for their antibacterial qualities; the Romans probably got these from the Egyptians who had used them for centuries.

Drug makers created dried ointment sticks, called *collyria*; these were short lengths of pre-mixed ingredients that a doctor could easily carry and then dissolve in water, milk, or egg white to make a usable salve. The collyria were usually marked with a stamp to identify the manufacturer. Archaeologists have discovered about 300 of these collyrium stamps, which usually contain the name of the disease, the name of the salve, and a person's name, probably the inventor of the salve or the maker of the medicine—the world's first brand-name drugs.

The great demand for rare herbs and spices from the East needed for botanical remedies gave rise to quack doctors and druggists who took advantage of a gullible public eager for cures. Galen—the Greek doctor practicing in Rome—obtained herbs directly from the emperor's own suppliers to ensure their genuineness. In Syria, he bought balsam of Mecca, and from a passing caravan on the Indian trade route, he purchased lycium, a tannin-rich extract highly effective in treating eye diseases.

CONTRACEPTION

Many different physicians had their own methods and formulas for birth control. In discussing contraception, Pliny says "Gossip records a miracle: that to rub juniper all over the male part before coitus prevents conception." Juniper is a strong uterine stimulator that can cause uterine tissue to contract and potentially cause contraception or spontaneous abortion. He warns that pregnant women must take care to exclude rue and water mint from their diet, because they may cause abortion. To induce sterility, Pliny recommends parsley and ferns.

Aetius of Amida, who lived in the sixth century AD, also mentions some male contraceptives. A man should rub alum, pomegranate, or oak galls with vinegar on his penis and he will not fertilize a woman. He even gives an oral contraceptive for men: the burned testicles of castrated mules drunk with a decoction of willow. For women, Aetius recommends a mixture of aloes, stock seeds, pepper, and saffron in wine. He also considered very effective an amulet made of a lioness's uterus placed in an ivory tube.

INDIA

AYURVEDA

Ancient India is one of the few places in the world that developed a coherent medical system whose tenets remain in practice today. Ayurvedic medicine is still practiced throughout the Indian subcontinent and is enjoying a burgeoning popularity in the West. In the ancient Indian language Sanskrit, Ayurveda means "the science of longevity" and is sometimes translated more broadly as "the science of life." The system seeks to restore harmony and balance to the body, mind, and spirit through a system of diet, herbal medicine, massage, purification, and lifestyle discipline.

In Ayurvedic medicine, the patient is active in his or her own preventative therapy. In this sense, Ayurveda is much more concerned with health than with disease—with the healthy person rather than with the unhealthy patient. Although one of the features that makes Ayurveda so popular today is its "holistic" approach, the truth is Ayurvedic medicine is firmly grounded in empirical observation and scientific theory. And while its ancient development and practice are not entirely devoid of magical charms and incantations, some of the earliest treatises on Ayurveda are remarkably rational and scientific.

DIVERSE BEGINNINGS

Scholars of Indology cannot determine the exact origins of Ayurveda, but we can see how many different traditions combined to create it over the millennia. The magical, religious lore of early Indian civilizations, the more empirical and practical approach of the so-called wandering ascetics, the medical traditions of the early Buddhist monks, and possible additions from neighboring traditions all work together to provide the basis of what we know as Ayurveda.

Out of these traditions emerges a system eventually codified in the two great Ayurvedic medical treatises—*Caraka Samhita* and *Susruta Samhita*. Although these two works, which provide the basis for the entire system, are considered Hindu, the information in them clearly developed over the centuries with significant help from the Buddhists and other religious and secular traditions.

BRAHMANISM

The sacred scriptures of Brahmanism are known as the Vedas. Chanted in Sanskrit and eventually written down, this work is a mixture of prose and verse, the oldest being poetry similar to hymns or psalms. Initially three books—the

Rgveda, the *Yajurveda*, and the *Samaveda*—made up the sacred scripture. The *Rgveda* and *Samaveda* are sacred poetry; the *Yajurveda* contains prose hymns devoted to sacrificial ritual. All three were primarily for the use of the Brahmans, or priestly class. However, a fourth book was later added to the triad: the *Atharvaveda*. This was the book of the atharvans—the magicians skilled in the art of fire and magic. Unlike the very sacred first three Vedas, which were intended for the Brahmans, the fourth book gave advice to the householder by way of spells, incantations, and magical charms useful for a host of problems, including medical conditions.

MEDICINE IN THE VEDAS

In addition to their spiritual significance, the Vedas also contain many references to medicine and healing. Vedic society viewed disease as a result of diabolical conditions and looked to healers to exorcize through magic, ritual, and herbal medicines the spirits that inhabited the sick person's body. Some medical references exist in the *Rgveda*, but they're mainly hymns to the healing deities the Ashvin twins (known as the "physicians of the gods") or to gods and goddesses that personify aspects of nature. A better source for medical information is the *Atharvaveda*.

The diseases discussed in the *Atharvaveda* can be divided into three types:

1. internal ailments caused by unseen sources
2. external afflictions brought on by injury or insect infestation, which include broken bones, loss of blood or hair, skin disorders, or flesh wounds
3. those illnesses caused by poisoning, which manifest themselves both internally and externally

Treating the diseases was again a matter of using the proper incantation from the *Atharvaveda*. In general, the *Atharvaveda* separates chants and incantations into two divisions—*bheshaja* (that which cures) and *adhichara* (sorcery). The bheshaja chants cover everything of a healing, medicinal nature—cures for fever, leprosy, jaundice, dropsy, and difficult childbirth. It also adds love charms and incantations to secure wealth, good fortune, and virility. There's even a spell to put an entire household to sleep so a lover can slip into the house undetected and join his beloved!

Adhichara spells bring bad luck or illness to one's enemies. A woman might, on occasion, cast a spell on a rival to make her a spinster forever or seek to destroy the virility of a man who had done her wrong. Replete with black magic and sorcery, adhichara spells provided hymns of praise to demons and serpents to garner their favor.

THE BHISHAJ

Medical practitioners in Vedic culture were called the *bhishaj* and their methods were derived principally from the *Atharvaveda*. It was the job of the bhishaj to rid his patient of disease. This might entail anything from exorcizing the disease demons from inside the body to mending a broken bone. Much like the shamans of earlier Indus Valley civilizations, the bhishaj understood medicinal plants, knew the proper spells and incantations, and, if necessary, could go into trances. He would use amulets and talismans made of plants and animal horns or burn a fragrant plant to ward off an evil spirit or to prepare the healing site. He also used water, which consistently offered healing properties for many diseases.

Divine Intervention. No matter what plant, fragrance, or surgical procedure the bhishaj used, the cure invariably came from the specific magical use of mantras, or spells. Reciting the proper hymns, using the correct incantation, invoking the right deity all gave power to the plant—and to the bhishaj—to cure an illness. Although it can't be known for sure, the bhishaj may have called upon the Ashvin twins for help when problems were serious. Likewise, he might invoke the particular god or goddess controlling the illness or the demon causing the problem in the first place. For example, if a patient suffered from dropsy, the bhishaj might invoke princely Varuna, the ruler of the waters, or call on Barahindevi, the demoness who caused the disease.

Transference. The bhishaj would sometimes rid the patient of a disease by transferring it to an animal, plant, or even a stone. He could do this in one of two ways: He could either manufacture a replica of the animal or plant by making one from wood or clay or choose another living entity for the transference. If he chose a replica, he would transfer the disease to it by using specific incantations and spells, and then he would throw it away or bury it. The living animal that received the disease by transference was driven away from the area or drowned, whereas a plant was burned.

Healing Substances. The *Atharvaveda* mentions several classifications of medical substances. Under the heading of animal substances, a bhishaj might choose rotten fish, animal saliva, tooth scorings, feathers, insects, frogs, or lice. There were various plants at his disposal and he used every part of its substance: the flower, root, leaves, thorns, bark, seeds, fruit, and sap. There is even mention in the *Atharvaveda* of using mineral substances to heal, including gold, silver, stones, and salt. The bhishaj always took great care in how he harvested his medicine; some of the rules make good botanical sense and others are incomprehensible. The ground in which the plant grew must be free of molds and large animal burrows or holes; the harvester must pick it while facing north and never use a weapon of war to cut it down. The plant itself must be healthy, devoid of blemishes, rot, and insect contamination.

Anatomy. Although the bhishaj was often called on to perform primitive surgery, he never possessed more than a superficial knowledge of anatomy. This was not because such information was lacking. Indeed, the Vedic scriptures contain very precise anatomical instructions. However, anatomy lessons remained the privilege of the priestly class, the Brahmans, and even they only really knew the anatomy of animals. Such knowledge was to be used only with sacrificial rituals. During sacrifices, priests had to be familiar with anatomical parts because as they butchered the animal, they recited the name of each body part and tossed a ball of rice into the sacred fire.

The Pariah. Although society looked on the bhishaj as a part of the community, he was not considered pure enough to join in sacrificial rituals. Since bhishaj was not a religious position, they remained outside the circle of priests, barred from ceremonial sacrifice.

VEDIC CURES

It is difficult to know the exact prescriptions that the bhishaj used, but the *Kausika Sutra*, written around the third century BC, is a treatise in the tradition of the *Atharvaveda* and gives us some picture of what early Vedic medicine might have been like:

akshata (tumor)—Tickle the area with the hair of a bull's tail; rub with dirt from the roots of a neem tree.

kasa (cough)—Drink clarified butter (ghee) in which dog's hair has been boiled.

kilasa (skin rashes)—Rub the area with a mixture of dog saliva and bull urine.

pakshabhata (paralysis)—Rub entire body with earth from inside the footprint of a dog; rub affected area with the ashes of an insect taken from a dog.

takman (fever)—Tie a frog to the leg of the patient's bed with red thread.

The Brahman class knew that the bhishaj traveled far and wide, healing the sick. Many patients were non-Aryans and, therefore, looked on as impure. The bhishaj himself was also considered impure and tainted to the Brahman not only because he associated with and cured inferior human beings but because in doing so he came into contact with polluted bodily fluids. Choosing to surround himself with the sick and the dying didn't help matters. A bhishaj could never quite be relegated to the status of an outcast, however, because he performed a necessary service. Even then, it didn't matter how you felt about doctors; you still needed them. A verse of the Rgveda explains it this way:

A poet who is a poet, physician, and apothecary in one person travels around the country carrying with him a wooden box full of all sorts of healing herbs and practicing his profession, not without humor and with a frankness that deserves recognition. He does not hide the fact that it is not philanthropy that motivates his practice, but that his main inspiration is gain.

THE WANDERING ASCETICS—
THE SRAMANAS

While Brahmanism was still dominant and the bhishajs were working their magic, another cultural movement was emerging that would change the face of healing in India. For ages, asceticism—the practice of self-denial and spiritual self-discipline—was revered in India. Ascetics were wanderers—spiritually and literally—and although they were never shunned, it can be said that they lived on the fringes of society, certainly not in the mainstream. In the sixth century BC, many of these ascetics were adherents to the nascent ascetic religions of Buddhism, Ajivika, and Jainism. It seems that at least some were well versed in the healing arts, and because they traveled extensively, exchanging ideas with other ascetics about what works and what doesn't, they soon developed an impressive array of therapeutics.

These wandering ascetics were called *sramanas*, or "strivers." Although some of the Vedic bhishaj could be numbered among the sramanas, the medical practices of the sramanas generally offered an empirical, less magical, view of healing; the ascetic healers relied on observation to diagnose and treat illness. They prescribed certain foods to cure internal diseases and applied plant-based poultices for external injuries. Unlike their bhishaj brethren, the sramanas did not believe in charging for their services. As "strivers," the sramanas were more concerned with the accumulation of knowledge rather than material gain; their path to understanding was based largely on experience. Because they did not ascribe to the taboos of their Brahman counterparts, they could entertain an interest in human anatomy.

They believed that humans were the epitome of nature. Theirs was, in truth, a philosophy of humanity. In fact, one of the ways in which a Buddhist ascetic contemplated impermanence and sought enlightenment was to meditate on a decomposing human body, focusing on every aspect not only externally—on hair, skin, bones, and teeth—but internally as well—on the blood, bile, liver, kidneys, spleen, and heart. They even meditated on bodily discharges. Although this direct scrutiny of a corpse—either in the mind or in the flesh—and meditation on bodily processes had more to do with religious observance than with medical research, it gave the ascetics a better understanding of the internal and external structures of the human body.

BUDDHIST INFLUENCE

Perhaps no other culture influenced the early medical lore that was to become Ayurveda more than the Buddhist monks. The knowledge the sramanas shared made up a rich tradition of healing, though nothing was written down or collected in any systematic way. About the middle of the fifth century BC, many Buddhist ascetics began to organize into spiritual communities called *sanghas.* Membership in these sanghas was open, and the monks encouraged other wanderers to seek shelter there. Visiting ascetics, eager to debate and exchange information, brought new ideas and healing strategies, which they debated with apparently great devotion.

MEDICINES

In later sangha life, monks were given five basic medicines—clarified butter, fresh butter, oil, honey, and molasses. At first, a patient was only allowed to consume these medicines twice a day—no more frequently than taking meals. In the Buddhist tradition, monks were not allowed to have any food after midday. According to the Buddhist scripture *Vinaya*, when Buddha discovered that some of the monks were not getting better, he decreed that these medicines could be administered more frequently. When he learned that these five cures still didn't do the job all the time, he added more medicines into the pharmacopoeia: roots, extracts, fruits, gums or resins, leaves, fats, and salts. These medicines, although food and plant based, could never be used to satisfy hunger—only to cure.

DOSHAS AND THE UNDERSTANDING OF DISEASE

As the sangha population stabilized, the monks and nuns began to standardize and codify all the medical information they had gathered. Much of this material can be found in the *Vinaya Pitaka* of the Buddhist Pali Canon, devoted to the code of conduct for the Buddhist monk.

The chapter on medicine represents the earliest form of Buddhist healing and closely parallels some of the information that would later be set down in the *Caraka Samhita* and the *Susruta Samhita*. Once written, this Buddhist "order of things" became the first step toward an Indian medical system. The Buddha identified the causes of disease as falling into one of the following categories:

- a change of season
- past actions (*karma*)
- unusual or excessive activities
- violent, external actions (being robbed or attacked)

Sramanic and Buddhist healers believed that humans represent or reflect the whole of nature—a belief also found in the Vedas. In other words, humans are microcosms of the universe, containing the same elements that make up all of creation. These elements—space (or ether), air, fire, water, and earth—are combined into three biological forces, or *doshas*, in humans—*vata, pitta,* and *kapha.*

- Vata is space and air.
- Pitta is fire and water.
- Kapha is water and earth.

The doshas came to be seen as responsible for all the functions of our bodies and minds. English has no adequate translation for the word *dosha*. Although you'll often see them referred to as air, fire, and water, respectively, or (less delicately) wind, bile, and phlegm, the concept of the dosha is more than that; for example, vata has wind-like qualities, but it is not simply wind.

The Buddhist canon, and later Ayurvedic medicine, views disease as a disruption of the doshas. Each dosha has its own seat, where it naturally resides in the body. Disruption of the dosha—its migration to, and accumulation in, another part of the body—will cause illness. For example, if vata is unseated from its seat in the lower bowels and moves to, say, the joints, arthritic symptoms may appear. It would be, therefore, the job of the medical practitioner to evaluate the problem and prescribe a treatment to rid the joints of excess vata.

Vata. Vata comes from the Sanskrit word *vayu*, meaning "wind," and indicates movement. Made up of air and ether, vata governs everything in the body that pertains to movement: blinking of the eyes, pulsations of the heart, and movement of the muscles. Its primary site in the body is the colon in the lower digestive tract, but it's also found below the navel in the thighs, hips, pelvis, bone marrow, bladder, large intestines, and nervous system. It governs the sense of touch. In the brain or nervous system, vata is responsible for anxiety, nervous energy, fear, and muscle spasms, as well as adaptability and comprehension. When vata accumulates, a person can suffer from flatulence, nervous disorders, insomnia, and confusion.

Pitta. Pitta is made up of fire and water. Located in the small intestines, blood, lymph, lower stomach, liver, spleen, eyes, skin, sweat, and sweat glands, pitta's fire controls digestion, absorption, assimilation, nutrition, bodily warmth, thirst, hunger, intelligence, and courage. Its primary site in the body is the stomach and the small intestines. Pitta brings about jealousy, anger, and hatred, as well as compassion, understanding, and perception. Excessive pitta causes inflammation, infections, indigestion, and jaundice.

Kapha. Kapha means phlegm. This dosha, composed of water and earth, denotes stability and solidity. Although its primary seat is in the lungs, kapha is also found in other parts of the upper body—the chest, throat, sinuses, head, upper stomach, fat tissues, nose, and the areas between the joints. It is responsible for maintaining lubrication and the body's immunity, strength, and sexual power. It keeps the skin moist, helps wounds heal, and provides energy to the heart and lungs. Its sense of calm and stability keeps vata and pitta under control. Kapha elicits avarice, greed, and attachment, as well as love, patience, and forgiveness. When kapha accumulates, a person suffers from excess mucus, swelling, nausea, lethargy, asthma, and depression.

An Individual's Constitution. Each one of these doshas by itself and in combination with the others is vital to the health of the body. Without vata, for example, kapha and pitta could not move. Kapha, which is part water, keeps vata from fanning the fire of pitta out of control and burning up the bodily tissues. Without pitta's fire, the digestive process could not take place.

Each person is made up of a unique combination of vata, pitta, and kapha. This combination, created at conception from the combined doshic makeup of one's parents, is called the *prakriti*, or constitution. To preserve good health, a person must maintain the same ratio of doshas he had when he was conceived. As a person grows up and responds to daily stresses and environmental changes, his or her doshas are stimulated and move. The predominant dosha is generally the one that fluctuates the most, so knowing the patient's doshic makeup is the first step in diagnosing any health problems. When a particular prakriti is out of balance, symptoms resulting from an excess dosha or a combination of doshas will manifest themselves. By understanding a person's doshic makeup, a physician can help anticipate potential problems before they arise and more accurately assess the nature of an illness when it occurs.

Rarely does a person have a predominance of only one dosha, although it is possible. Besides the monotype vata, pitta, and kapha constitutions, there are the duotype combinations of vata-pitta, pitta-kapha, vata-kapha, and the very rare tri-doshic vata-pitta-kapha, sometimes called *sama*.

Vata Types. Remembering that vata is the dosha composed of air and space, it is apparent that vata personality types tend to be fast-talkers, quick-thinkers, and have extreme characteristics—very tall with protruding joints and bones and dry, rough skin. Motion through space (mentally and physically) characterizes vatas, who go unburdened. No excess weight gets in their way—they are generally thin and wiry. Since air (or wind) dries out whatever it comes into contact with, vata types may suffer from digestive problems such as constipation—there's not enough lubrication to loosen things. They don't always take the time to eat, and their appetite varies. Mentally, vata types move at a rapid pace. With no time to sit around and ponder, they grasp concepts readily, have thousands of ideas every minute, and possess a creative, active imagination. Unfortunately, they often forget things almost as quickly as they grasp them and have trouble putting their ideas into practice. In business, they make great brainstormers and, with a characteristic generous nature, can spur coworkers on to great things.

Pitta Types. Pitta, on the other hand, is ruled by fire primarily. Unlike the element of air that flits from one place to another, fire is rooted in one place and burns steady and long. The heat of fire in itself can dry things out. Fueled by fire, pitta types have a strong metabolism and can digest their foods readily, but they can suffer from acid indigestion from a digestive system that's too aggressive. Pitta types tend to be thin and delicate, though not to the extreme of their vata brethren.

Mentally, pitta types share some traits with vata types. Like vatas, they master concepts quickly, enjoy a lot of activity, and are very intelligent. However, with their fire aspect burning steadily, pitta types have no trouble concentrating on the task at hand. They enjoy the challenge of working through a problem, and their good, quick memory comes in handy. In business, pittas make good planners and have the staying power to see those plans through. Their fiery dispositions, however, cause them to be short-tempered and quick to jump to conclusions; pittas are hotheads.

Kapha Types. Water and earth govern the kapha dosha. The qualities of water (lubricating, cool, and shapeless) and earth (heavy, inert, dry, calm, and solid) show up in people with predominantly kapha personalities. These "salt-of-the-earth" types tend to have well-developed physiques and strong appetites.

Mentally, kapha personalities exhibit the characteristics of both water and earth. They are calm, even-tempered, loving, dependable, and forgiving. Unlike vatas, whose beliefs change with the wind, and pittas, whose convictions are extremely strong and passionate, kaphas exhibit deep, solid beliefs that don't change readily. In business, they are loyal and dependable organizers.

THE EMERGENCE OF AYURVEDA

By the first few centuries AD, Hinduism was once again ascendant in India. Buddhism found adherents to the east in Tibet and China, and Hinduism absorbed a great deal of theology and science from the Buddhists. In medicine as religion, the Hindus incorporated what they valued from the Buddhist tradition into their emerging system. Elaborating on earlier concepts and finally codifying what was probably common, orally transmitted knowledge, Indian physicians were finally setting down the tenets of Ayurveda.

THE SAMHITAS

The *Caraka Samhita* and *Susruta Samhita*, the sacred medical texts, represent the first true codification of the Ayurvedic system. The *Caraka Samhita* is primarily a clinical medical text; the *Susruta Samhita* is primarily a surgical text. The *Samhitas* make up the basis of Ayurveda and are still considered authoritative on many issues today.

It's hard to say exactly when the *Samhitas* were written down. Some scholars say the *Caraka Samhita* dates from the second century AD and the *Susruta* from the fourth. It's also likely that both works represent a compilation of data that spans several centuries, beginning a few hundred years BC. What we do know is that both texts include medical information from the early wandering physicians as well as revisions added during a much later era to incorporate Hindu medical lore. The later Hindu, or Brahmanic, additions (around the fourth or fifth century AD) reflect a desire to justify the art of healing and incorporate it into their religious tradition—the tradition of the Vedas.

Although the Buddhist monk-healers prided themselves on using only the most empirical and rational means to cure the sick, magic never truly disappeared from the Indian medical scene. The *Samhitas* do, in fact, contain some magical and religious doctrines, showing that the Vedic culture of the bhishaj still had a strong hand in Indian medicine despite the influence of the Buddhists' more scientific approach. The *Caraka Samhita* recognizes its power to heal and defines "divine source" as one of the three forms of therapy. It explains that sometimes a physician needs to resort to reciting mantras, using amulets, making fire offerings, invoking the name of certain deities, or embarking on a pilgrimage to rid his patient of a tenacious disease. Despite the presence of some magical charms and a general gloss of Brahmanic religion, the two texts are still mainly scientific treatises. They continue and expand the work of the Buddhists, recording more classifications as well as giving specific diagnoses and treatments.

The Gunas. In the *Samhitas*, this concept is best exemplified by the three *gunas*. According to one of the earliest of the orthodox philosophies of Hinduism, the primordial energy involved in creation was made up of three distinct attributes or gunas—*sattva* (goodness or essence), *rajas* (movement or passion), and *tamas* (darkness or inertia). The interaction of these three attributes caused the evolution of the universe. The gunas—sattva, rajas, and tamas—create all existence as we know it, and also manifest themselves as emotional and mental predispositions that make up our character.

Sattva, or essence, expresses goodness, compassion, and clarity. Generally, sattvic people are charitable, intelligent, religious, strong, and courageous. Sattvic foods are easy to digest and generally bland—milk, clarified butter (ghee), wheat, and certain fruits and vegetables.

Rajas suggests passion, movement, transformation, and aggressiveness. Rajastic people tend to be good in business dealings, forceful, political, and extroverted. Taken to an extreme, they can suffer from jealousy and selfishness. Rajastic foods include meat (except beef) and fish and can be salty, pungent, and bitter.

Tamas denotes inertia, gloom, darkness, and laziness. A person who is overly tamasic is dull, slow-witted, and selfish. It drives sexual energy and material desires. Tamasic foods include onions and garlic, beef, alcohol, and mushrooms.

The Elements. The five gross elements of ether, air, fire, water, and earth that make up the external universe and inorganic matter manifest in our bodies as the senses—hearing, touching, seeing, tasting, and smelling. They help us perceive the world in which we live.

Ether, or space, enables the ear to function and manifests as sound. It is light, cool, elastic, mobile, and exists everywhere. Sound expresses itself through speech, so the ear and the mouth are connected.

Air relates to the skin and manifests as touch. The hand is the organ of action, enabling the body to experience the tangible world, through giving, holding, and receiving. It is not only light and cool like ether, but dry and clear as well.

Fire enables the eye to see, bringing color and form to the forefront. It is hot, dry, and bright, with upward movement, and it manifests as sight. The sense of sight also connects to walking, giving the walker a sense of direction. Therefore, fire is also related to the feet, and controls movement.

Water is the element of taste and of the tongue. Its attributes are liquid, cold, and downward movement.

Earth is the element of smell and the nose. It is heavy, rough, inert, and hard. The function of the nose closely relates to the excretory action of the anus and therefore controls elimination.

AGNI: THE FIRE INSIDE

The *Caraka Samhita* introduces the concept of *grahani*, the seat of digestive fire, or *agni*. This internal organ "seizes" the food and releases the power of the fire. Located above the navel, this phantom organ, according to Caraka: "checks undigested food and releases the digested [food] from the side; but when the digestive fire is weak, it [the grahani] becomes defective and gives off undigested food." In Ayurveda, agni governs metabolism, breaking down the food we eat and turning it into energy and waste products that we can absorb and eliminate. Of course, there's more than one agni in the body; in fact there are 13 of them.

THE THREE MALAS

Vital to health in Ayurveda is proper elimination of the three *malas* or waste products—feces, urine, and sweat. Urine and feces form during digestion, so it's imperative that agni, the digestive fire, works optimally. Ayurveda sees a connection between sweat and urination, which are both pitta-related and reduce water content in the body. Modern Ayurvedic physicians believe diabetes, dropsy, and skin diseases such as psoriasis result from an accumulation of pitta in the skin, causing it to be out of balance with the kidneys.

THE SEVEN DHATUS

The *dhatus* loosely correspond to the body's tissues and fluids. They are responsible for the entire structure of the body. The order of the dhatus is especially important. The health of a particular dhatu depends on the health of the previous one since each dhatu is formed and receives its nourishment from the one before it. Here are the dhatus in serial order:

1. **Rasa—plasma and lymph.** Sanskrit for "sap" or "juice," rasa includes tissue fluids, chyle, lymph, and plasma and contains all the nutrients from digested food. Rasa, which circulates through the body with the help of the vata dosha, serves to nourish all tissues, organs, and systems in the body. Governed by kapha, rasa's byproducts include menstruation blood and breast milk. Rasa flows from the heart through 24 ducts—10 going up, 10 going down, and 4 going sideways—feeding the whole body. It takes five days to convert rasa into blood and a month to transmute it into sperm or ova.

2. **Rakta—blood.** More than just the blood that flows through the body, rakta, which comes from rasa, serves to invigorate the system and maintain life. Its action is governed by pitta. Ancient Ayurvedic physiology believed that a disruption of pitta, therefore, spoils the blood and makes it black, blue, frothy, green, too slow or too fast, and toxic.

3. **Mamsa—muscle and flesh.** Including all the muscle tissue, tendons, and flesh that cover the body's organs, mamsa functions to stabilize the system. Connected with the element earth and the kapha dosha, mamsa controls the movement of the joints and maintains the body's strength. Mamsa is simply blood heated by agni (fire) and condensed by vata (the bodily winds).

4. **Meda—fat.** Oily and kapha (water and earth) by nature, fat works to "oil" the system and keep the tissues lubricated. Meda is mamsa (or flesh) further transformed and deposited under the skin and under the belly.

5. **Asthi—bone.** This dhatu gives support to the whole system and includes bone and cartilage. Governed by air and earth, asthi is meda (fat) heated by the natural fires (agni) and dried by the bodily winds (vata) until it hardens.

6. **Majjan—marrow and nerve tissue.** The bone marrow is what the ancient texts referred to as the "oily perspiration of the bones," and includes red and yellow marrow. This "oily perspiration" congeals to fill in the spaces between the bones. Majjan also carries motor and sensory impulses to the brain.

7. **Shukra—reproductive.** According to Ayurveda, shukra originates from the bone marrow and contains the ingredients of all tissues. Concentrated in the reproductive organs, shukra includes male and female sexual fluids and governs

reproduction and immune functions. Shukra comes from the bone marrow and produces the essence Ayurveda calls *ojas*—a substance difficult to translate, but loosely described as vitality or bodily strength.

THE SROTAS

The physical body produces nutrients it must transport to its various tissue sites and waste products it has to expel. To do this, it needs avenues to transport them all. These avenues or channels are called *srotas*. There are 13 of them: big channels with large passageways (large and small intestines and the uterus, for example); small channels with narrow passageways (blood vessels); and subtle channels that don't appear to have any physical opening but that allow for transportation anyway (nerves). Improper flow as well as excessive buildup of doshas in any of these channels causes disease.

THE PICTURE OF HEALTH

Good health means that the entire body is working efficiently. The mind discriminates effectively when the three gunas of balance, energy, and inertia (sattva, rajas, tamas) are in equilibrium. The body is healthy when:

- the digestive fire (agni) is burning properly
- the three doshas are working together optimally
- the seven dhatus are functioning properly
- the 13 srotas are open and flowing properly
- the three malas—urine, feces, and sweat—are efficiently eliminated

In other words, everything must function in harmony. When everything is in tune, the immune system can then offer natural resistance even to contagious diseases, and a person's mental and emotional health will be strong.

CLASSIFICATION OF DISEASE

The earliest Ayurvedic texts identify disease in terms of an eight-fold classification system. The Buddhists attributed four of the eight causes to doshic disruption (vata, pitta, kapha, and a combination of the three). The other four causes included changes of season, stressful or unusual activities, violent or traumatic events, and past actions (karma). But Ayurvedic medicine divides the eight-limbed system into three broader categories. *Adhyatmika* takes into account the four doshic imbalances and karma; *adhibhautika* includes stressful activities and violent events; *adhidaivika* includes the change of seasons and supernatural causes. Although adhidaivika is somewhat contrary to early Buddhist medical doctrine, it reflects early Ayurveda's unwillingness to let go of the magical and religious causes of disease completely.

Ayurveda equates all disease with doshic disruption, without negating the age-old premise that disease stems from internal, external, and unexplained causes. It simply says that everything in the universe has doshic properties. These properties and the way in which a person interacts with his or her environment can affect health: the food eaten, attitudes held, the people associated with, the time of year, and even the time of day. In other words, a person's internal environment constantly interacts with the environment around him. When the two are out of balance, a person gets sick.

INTERNAL FACTORS

Weak digestive agni prevents food from being broken down properly, causing it to remain in the system. This undigested or improperly digested mass accumulates in the srotas, blocks them, and putrefies into a sticky substance called *ama*. Ama is basically made up of undigested or improperly digested food and any external toxins the body cannot expel. Ayurveda considers the accumulation of ama to be one of the major causes of disease. Symptoms of ama accumulation are a coated tongue, bad breath, headaches, body odor, and a general feeling of heaviness. Not having been broken down properly, ama is thick and dense, so it ends up clogging the channels, preventing them from contributing to the formation of the subsequent channels.

Diseases from ama accumulation vary according to the three doshas. This is to say, an Ayurvedic physician must take into account which dosha-ama is dominant so as to determine how to treat the resultant disease. A kapha-ama condition, for example, will manifest as indigestion and congestion with thick mucus that is difficult to expel. A pitta-ama (toxic fire) condition also manifests as indigestion with the addition of fever and diarrhea. Vata-ama (toxic air) conditions bring indigestion, bloating, constipation, gas, and arthritis.

Another internal factor can be depleted *ojas*. Ojas—the essential energy produced by the seventh dhatu—gives vitality and health to the body and mind. When ojas is reduced, disease follows. Diseases that stem from low ojas generally are difficult to cure and include most infectious and nervous disorders.

Negative or repressed emotions, according to Ayurveda, can also contribute to ill health. All emotions (present or the results of past karma) remain imprinted in our muscles and certain organs and correspond to particular doshas. Repressed anger, for example, aggravates pitta, changing the balance of the gallbladder, bile duct, and small intestines. Ayurveda recommends that emotions never be held inside.

EXTERNAL FACTORS

The most common external factors affecting health are diet, environmental toxins, and lifestyle stress. Ayurveda also understands that the passage of time affects the body's ability to stay balanced. Eating at the right time, going to bed by a certain hour, pacifying the body at the right month of the year, all have beneficial effects on a person's health.

Dietary Factors. There's a Western adage that aptly describes the Ayurvedic understanding of food: "You are what you eat." What a person puts into his or her body and how the body responds to and digests it can adversely or positively affect health. Certain foods aggravate certain doshas. For example, popcorn, which is dry and full of air, doesn't digest well in a person whose vata is out of balance. It can cause bloating and excess gas. Kaphas who feel sluggish and possessive should stay away from kapha foods such as ice cream, avocados, or winter squash. Pittas, especially in the heat of the summer, should refrain from adding hot chili peppers or onions to their food.

Planetary Influences. The ancient healers believed that the planets and other heavenly spheres influenced the body and, particularly, the mind of human beings. Physicians sometimes asked the patient to have his or her astrologic chart read, or they would interpret his or her dreams to pinpoint the exact cause and placement of the disease.

Biological Time. Childhood, adulthood, and old age are all ruled internally by the doshas. Kapha governs the first 16 years of life. During infancy, a child depends on her mother's milk for sustenance; later childhood years are marked with kapha-like diseases: colds, flu, congestion, and ear infections. Throughout these years, children are growing and developing strong tissues, and their bodies need constant nourishment. Adulthood lasts until age 55 and is governed by pitta. These are the most active, vital years of a person's life. When pitta is out of control, teenagers tend to suffer from acne and older adults get digestive disorders. Vata controls the later years. This is the time when metabolism slows and tissues are not replenished as readily. Vata disorders in old age include arthritis, poor memory, tremors, and wrinkles.

Chronologic Time. The doshas also govern chronologic time. Early morning belongs to kapha. It's a time of awakening, stretching, and beginning the day. A person may feel somewhat heavy, slower than other times during the day, but fresh and alert. Midday is pitta time—when the digestive juices start flowing and a person gets hungriest. This is the time of day when Ayurvedic practitioners would recommend having the main meal of the day, when the digestive agni is at its peak. In the afternoon, vata takes over. This is the time of activity and high energy. In the evening, kapha comes back. This, according to Ayurveda, is the time to slow down, relax, and prepare for sleep. Pitta kicks in again around 10 p.m. and works to digest the day's food until 2 a.m. when vata resurfaces. Vata time—between 2 a.m. and 6 a.m.—is the time for dreaming and beginning the process of awakening. Ayurveda believes a person should wake up before 6 a.m. when vata is still active so that he or she can arise refreshed and energized, and so that elimination of waste products will happen easily.

Seasonal Time. Knowing the aspects of the three doshas, it's easy to see how they are related to the seasons. The autumn months through early winter—a time of windy days and falling temperatures—are a vata time. With winter in full swing, plant life dies, animals migrate to warmer climes, and people come down with colds and other upper respiratory ailments. This is the time of kapha, ruler of the lungs and the dosha of water and earth. The transition between winter and spring still sees the influence of kapha as the effects of winter begin to thaw—snow melts, the earth softens, animals give birth. As the earth and air heat up, pitta takes over. Late spring and summer bring a host of pitta–induced ailments like rashes, diarrhea, allergies, and sunburns.

DIAGNOSING DISEASE

Diagnosis takes on a much different meaning in Ayurveda than it does in Western medicine. Ayurvedic doctors prefer to monitor the body before illness is manifest. For thousands of years, Ayurvedic healers have relied on their keen powers of observation and their knowledge of the interactions of micro- and macro-anatomy to diagnose disharmony in the body. Through an elaborate interview process, urine and feces analysis, and observation of the tongue, skin, eyes, nails, and other physical features, Ayurvedic doctors can determine which doshas, tissues, channels, and organs are affected. To find the disturbed dosha, a physician needs to establish the patient's individual prakriti. An Ayurvedic physician takes into account a patient's mental and emotional condition as well.

When diagnosing an illness, according to the *Caraka Samhita*, a physician must take into account the following items:

- patient's condition
- family background, heredity, and caste
- climate, food, and water in the country of the patient's birth
- character and temperament
- physical constitution
- whether the disease is hot or cold

The *Caraka Samhita* also specifies the proper physical examination, which should include:

- general appearance of the patient
- the feel of the patient's skin (checking temperature)
- examination of eyes, tongue, feces, and urine
- tasting the secretions of the patient, when appropriate

An Ayurvedic physician observes the body with care. This ancient diagnostic tool is still relied on by physicians to give them the information they need. For instance, noticing that a person's skin is rough, cracked, or chapped, a physician could ascertain a vata imbalance. If a patient is hot to the touch and flush of face, a physician would diagnose a pitta imbalance; a pale, drawn complexion of a patient who feels cold would indicate aggravated kapha.

Face. A physician can tell a lot from a face. Ayurveda teaches that emotions can lodge in the tissues, most evidently in the face. Worry lines, bags under the eyes, and cheek discoloration all indicate general constitution as well as emotional state.

Eyes. The eyes are also good indicators of health and well-being. The eyes may be the windows to the soul, but they also provide another diagnostic tool for physical illness. The condition and coloration of the eyes, as well as any abnormalities, are indicative of a variety of problems.

Tongue. The doctor observes the size, shape, color, and contour of the tongue. If the tongue has a white coating on it, toxins may be present. If the tongue's coloring is pale, the patient could be anemic; a yellowish color indicates problems in the liver or gallbladder; a bluish cast points to heart problems.

Lips and Nails. The condition of both the lips and the nails can also help a physician ascertain an imbalance in the patient. Like the tongue, the physician pays attention to color and size. However, general appearance and consistency can be equally informative. A nutrient deficiency will cause white spots on nails; ridges indicate malabsorption, and, of course, bitten or torn nails can show that the patient is nervous or anxious.

Most Westerners are familiar with checking their pulses by putting their two fingers against the pressure points on either side of their wrists or throat. Persian healers probably introduced a much more elaborate system of pulse reading to Ayurveda around the fourteenth century. Physicians learned to read the pulses on the nose, neck, armpit, inner arm above the elbow, wrist, groin, and ankle to determine the strength or weakness of the pulse, its character, and the number of beats per minute. Pulse readings inform the practitioner as to disruptions of the doshas and even the presence or diminution of ojas, that untranslatable term we call life force, energy, or vitality.

URINE EXAMINATION

Like pulse diagnosis, urine examination as a diagnostic tool probably did not arrive in Ayurvedic circles until the thirteenth or fourteenth centuries. Color, clarity, consistency, and odor can indicate of doshic imbalances. Sometimes, the physician puts a drop of sesame oil into the urine sample and holds it up to the sunlight for inspection. If the drop diffuses quickly, the disease is easy to cure; if the drop sinks to the middle of the urine, the illness is more serious and difficult to cure; if the drop sinks all the way to the bottom, the disease is very difficult to treat. A physician can also tell from the urine sample what type of imbalance a patient suffers from. If the drop of sesame oil spreads in wavy patterns like a snake, too much vata is present; if the drop breaks up into colors like a rainbow pattern, pitta is indicated; if the oil drops like a pearl, it suggests a kapha imbalance.

TREATMENTS

Since all disease stems from a disruption in the doshas, treatment must begin to return the body to a state of doshic harmony. Ayurvedic physicians use diet, herbs, and cleansing techniques to counteract the manifestation of disease in the body. Ayurveda believes it is vital to eliminate the toxins that are causing the disease before attempting to pacify or temper the body. The reasons are simple: First, if a doctor prescribes a treatment that merely attends to the superficial symptoms of an ailment, the disease may go further into the tissues and move away from the treatment. So while the symptoms may get better temporarily, in the long run the disease will manifest elsewhere in the body, causing further debilitating symptoms. Second, an accumulation of undigested foods or toxins (ama) prevents the body from absorbing the herbs and foods designed to treat the disease.

There were and are several primary means of treatment to prepare or tone the body. To eliminate disease from the tissues, Ayurveda uses a two-step approach: palliation and purification. In a way, palliation therapy is similar to the Western-style approach called detoxification and cleansing. Purification therapy, however, goes beyond the Western understanding of elimination. Ayurveda believes no treatment can successfully eliminate the toxic wastes from the body without first directing these toxins to their proper channels of elimination. If disease manifests in the body because of an imbalance in the gastrointestinal tract (the first stage of disease), an Ayurvedic physician will almost always perform purification therapy. If the disease has already entered the tissues, however, palliation techniques must precede purification.

PALLIATION

Palliation means "to pacify." The herbs administered during this phase attempt to break up the toxins and calm the doshas enough to expel the excesses when purification therapy begins. The *Ashtanga Hridaya Samhita*, an Ayurvedic text from around the seventh century AD, explains how palliation therapy uses "herbs to burn up toxins, herbs to stimulate digestion, fasts, and exercise" to strengthen agni, the digestive fire, which in turn destroys the toxins.

Also called *purvakarma*, this treatment program can be administered by a doctor or sometimes by the sick person him- or herself. To loosen toxins and cleanse the body, the physician would use honey, clarified butter (ghee), long pepper (if the patient can't tolerate ghee), or sesame or castor oil.

PALLIATIVE THERAPY

Although palliative therapy can last from one week to a few months, one example of a short-term pitta-eliminating palliative therapy would be:

Day One: Take one tablespoon of ghee first thing in the morning followed by a cup of warm water. Drink several cups of warm water throughout the day. Eat lighter meals than normal.

Day Two: Take three tablespoons of ghee upon rising; drink several cups of warm water throughout the day. Eat lighter meals than normal.

Day Three: Take six tablespoons of ghee in the morning; drink several cups of warm water throughout the day. Eat lighter meals than normal.

Day Four: Take nine tablespoons of ghee in the morning; drink several cups of warm water throughout the day. Eat lighter meals than normal.

Day Five: Do not take any additional ghee. Drink warm water throughout the day. Eat light, preferably vegetarian meals.

Day Six: Take several capsules of senna leaf as a laxative. Do not eat any food until most of the cleansing has subsided.

Honey eliminates excess kapha; ghee, long pepper, or castor oil gets rid of pitta; and sesame oil eliminates vata. Purvakarma has to begin about five days to a week before purification therapy. Other palliative therapies include massage and heat, which are external treatments to cause the patient to relax or sweat.

PURIFICATION THERAPY

According to the *Ashtanga Hridaya Samhita*, "cleansing enemas, nasal medication, purgation, vomiting, and blood-letting," were the five methods of purification. These five actions were designed to rid the body completely and finally of the excessive doshas and ama causing an acute disease. If a patient is in a weakened condition, usually a physician modifies the panchakarma therapy, often leaving out the more severe methods.

Therapeutic Vomiting (vanuna). Generally the patient drinks three cups of a strong tea made from licorice root, salt, calamus root, or lobelia. If that doesn't work, a couple glasses of salt water first thing in the morning should do the trick. Physicians never prescribe vomiting for those who are weak, too old, too young, or who suffer from a hacking, dry cough.

Purgation Therapy (virecana). This therapy is used to rid the body of excess pitta from the small intestines, colon, kidneys, liver, and gallbladder. Purgation, or laxative, therapy treats constipation, diarrhea, dysentery, and food poisoning. Lots of different herbs are used as mild laxatives: castor oil, senna leaf, dandelion root, psyllium seed, cascara sagrada, and flaxseed husks.

Enema Therapy (basti). Enemas are used to rid the body of excess vata. Castor oil is sometimes used, but dry enemas are sometimes used with it in an alternating fashion.

Nasal Therapy (nasya). Ayurvedic physicians swear by nasal application of herbs. It works well for sinus conditions, dry coughs, scratchy throats, migraine headaches, and feelings of nervousness, anxiety, and fear. The physician places a few drops of herbal oil on his or her finger and inserts it as far into the nose as possible. Then the physician massages the nose, helping the medicated oil to reach far into the passages. The use of a *neti* pot is another form of nasal therapy. It involves pouring warm, salted water up one nostril and out the other.

Bloodletting (raktamokshana). Although not popular in the West, bloodletting is an ancient form of Ayurvedic treatment employing leeches to purify the blood. A gentler, effective method of purifying the blood is burdock root tea. A patient begins by clearing out the system with a gentle laxative. For the next two to three months, the patient then drinks burdock root tea every evening, allowing the action of the herb to purify and tonify the blood.

DIET

Besides prescribing purvakarma and panchakarma treatments, an Ayurvedic doctor takes care to monitor a patient's diet. There would be no use in going through an intensive series of elimination and tonifying treatments if the patient plans to return to a poor diet and an unhealthy lifestyle. All foods affect the doshic makeup of the individual, and it is critical to eat the foods that do not promote or exacerbate a doshic imbalance. For example, a person suffering from excess vata may feel dry, cold, nervous, and agitated. To eat foods that are also dry, cold, or bitter would only exacerbate the situation. So a physician would prescribe vata-suppressing foods such as seaweeds (formed from fire and water) that clean out the tissues or would prescribe sour foods such as miso and lemons that would aid digestion.

Physicians classify foods by taste (*rasa*), by potency (*virya*), by qualities or attributes (*guna*), and by aftertaste (*vipaka*). One popular Ayurvedic method of classifying food and medicine is by how they taste on the tongue: sweet, sour, bitter, pungent, salty, or astringent. Like the doshas, each taste, or rasa, corresponds to two of the five gross elements: Sweet comprises earth and water; sour is a combination of earth and fire; bitter combines air and ether; pungent comprises fire and air; salty combines water and fire; and astringent brings together earth and air.

With the understanding that "like increases like," it's easy to see how a physician would need to know the qualities of any medicine he or she would want to prescribe. A pitta imbalance, for example, may bring on an ulcer, result in excessive sweating, or create acidic urine, all of which point to too much heat in the body. The medicine prescribed would need to be cooling, dry, heavy, and dull (the opposite of pitta) to be effective.

Once the doctor determines the medical problem and its characteristics and attributes, it is time to choose and prepare the medicines for use. For the physician to use a medicine, it must pass several tests:

- Does it cure more than one disease?
- Will it treat the disease at its site of origin and at the site of manifestation?
- Can it prevent the disease from spreading any further?
- Can it be prepared in several ways to accommodate the patient's needs?
- Will it produce any adverse side effects?

Botanical Medicines. There are several ways to prepare the hundreds of botanicals Ayurveda uses as medicines, such as the following:

- Extractions are juice or sap extracted from plant parts.
- Infusions are plant parts or herbs steeped in boiling water.
- Decoctions are plants or herbs simmered in water until the water is reduced and the plant part softened.
- Powders, or *churnas*, are pulverized dried plant parts or herbs.
- Pastes, plasters, or oils are made from plant or herbal extracts, similar to the powders with the addition of a liquid. These were especially useful for external injuries such as sprains, broken bones, or joint problems.
- Herbally infused oils—sesame, coconut, sunflower, or olive—are used for enemas, massages, or dry or itchy scalp conditions.
- Pills or suppositories are herbs or plant extracts usually ground up and inserted into vegetable-based capsules or suppositories for internal use.
- Boluses are pulverized herbs or plant parts placed in a muslin sack, dipped in very warm water or milk, and rubbed over the body.
- Alcoholic extracts are herbs boiled then distilled or simply added to the alcohol.

Mineral Medicines. The use of minerals and metals is almost as old as Ayurveda itself. At least four types of medicines were prepared this way. The first are called sublimates, which are medicines made by sublimating sulphur (taking it from its solid state to a vapor quickly) in a glass container. The second group are called *bhasmas*, which are ash residues from metals, gems, plants, and animal by-products. Mercury is the most common bhasma and contributes to the increase of red blood cells. The third group, called *pishtis*, combine pulverized gems with juices and extracts. The fourth group of mineral-based medicines, *collyrium*, is the residue of antimony powder, lead oxide, or lamp soot mixed with castor oil and used to improve eyesight.

Tonics. After treating a particular ailment, a physician would often recommend tonics, or *rasayanas*, to keep the body functioning optimally. Rasayanas are herbal elixirs or tonics used to tone and strengthen the body's tissues and keep the doshas in balance. They promote longevity and youthfulness, two important goals of health in Ayurveda.

SURGERY

Surgical procedures were not foreign to Ayurvedic practitioners even in ancient times. Indeed, one of the two great *Samhitas* is a surgical text. The *Susruta Samhita* describes many types of surgery for tumors, bone fractures, dental problems, and eye diseases, among other conditions.

Some of the techniques were not uncommon in other parts of the ancient world—cautery, bloodletting, cupping—but some were well ahead of their time. Grafting of tissue was used to repair wounds and congenital defects. Susruta discusses the surgical repair of ears and noses damaged by accident or as a form of punishment. This type of advanced plastic surgery was not developed in the rest of the world for centuries.

Patient care before, during, and after the operation was not neglected. Preparatory measures—actually a form of *purvakarma*—included waiting for the astrologically auspicious moment and ensuring the proper deities were honored and all the surgical instruments were clean and within reach. During the surgical treatment (*pradhanakarma*), cold water sprayed on the face was used for the patient's pain, and the surgeon was instructed to move swiftly and surely so as not to prolong the procedure. Postoperative care (*pashcatkarma*) included such familiar modern procedures as observation in a special nursing chamber (a recovery room) and frequently changed wound dressings. The surgeons were acutely aware of the dangers of such procedures. Susruta carefully instructs the surgeon to keep instruments clean and sharp and even to apply alcoholic liquids to the incision site. Certain mortal points, or *marmans*, were to be avoided at all costs; these 107 marmans were areas where veins, arteries, or nerve bundles were particularly vulnerable to damage, with very serious repercussions. Wounds were constantly monitored for postoperative infections, and many poultices and other medicines were used to prevent them.

LIFESTYLES AND WELLNESS

Ayurveda firmly believes in preventative health care. Many physicians advocate panchakarma (purification) treatments at the change of each season, but certainly in the springtime. This helps clean out the system and prepare the body for the new season. They will caution that their patients pay particular attention to their diet and their daily routine, taking care to listen to their body's needs. Ayurvedic recommendations act as a reminder to stay in sync with the rhythms of the external world, which is also governed by the five gross elements—ether, air, fire, water, and earth—and, in turn, relate to the three do-shas—vata, pitta, and kapha. Only by maintaining this balance can we maintain health. If the biological balance is upset, Ayurveda can restore doshic harmony. Knowledge of the causes of illness, how it is manifested in the humors, and the tissues and pathways affected are crucial to maintaining this equilibrium.

YOGA

Yoga sees health as a state of bodily harmony that cannot be taken for granted and, as such, demands serious discipline. Falling ill usually denotes a false relationship to one's life and to other people. Feeling ill at ease or alienated from society contributes to creating disease in the body. To return to good health, a yogin must return to a moral and happy life, understanding his or her interconnectedness to all beings.

Yoga's rich history begins in India perhaps as early as 2000 BC. Although yoga did not develop as a codified system of philosophy until around the second century AD, there's evidence of yogic postures dating back to the Harappan culture of the Indus Valley.

Yogic techniques appear many times in the Upanishads, treatises that date back to between 800 and 500 BC. The authors of these mystical teachings believed that liberation came through knowledge. The word comes from the root *upa* meaning "near," *ni* which means "down," and *sad* meaning "to sit." This refers to the way in which the Upanishads were taught. The student sat down near his or her teacher, or guru, who, in turn, imparted the secret doctrines of these texts.

THE EARLY PHILOSOPHY OF YOGA

Much like the science of Ayurveda, yoga is based on Samkhya, one of the earliest Hindu philosophical systems; yoga added the notion of God, however, a concept not found in Samkhya. The two main categories of existence for Samkhya are *Purusha* (pure, transcendental spirit or self; male) and *Prakriti* (nature or matter; female). Purusha has no beginning and no end; it simply is. Prakriti, on the other hand, is dynamic, creative, and distinct; it is in constant motion. Prakriti creates three distinct manifestations of itself, called *gunas*. These manifestations exist at the same time, but in differing degrees, in everything that makes up the cosmos. An understanding of the three gunas helps to explain how each relates to existence:

Sattva—This guna manifests the mind and the five cognitive senses. The mind coordinates all biological and psychic activities and controls the subconscious. The cognitive senses (eyes, ears, nose, tongue, and skin) help us acquire knowledge and put us in touch with the external world.

Rajas—When rajas is in control, the senses of yearning manifest: the voice, hands, feet, anus, and genitals. Rajas makes motor energy and physical experience possible. It controls passion and the activity of the body.

Tamas—Tamas is darkness of consciousness. When this guna predominates, the five subtle elements appear. These are the *potentials* of sound, sight, taste, touch, and smell, which give rise to all structures.

According to the Samkhya system, suffering, disease, and confusion all come from the misguided understanding that the cosmos is real. Existence is, in fact, a manifestation of imbalance, just like disease is. In other words, when one guna predominates over the others, it gives rise to the appearance of phenomena, including the senses.

If a person becomes attached to phenomena or their effects, falsely believing that what he or she sees, hears, tastes, touches, or smells exists in and of itself, he or she becomes deluded. This delusion creates further attachments and confusion and pushes the person further away from the higher self. Yogic philosophy strives to keep the gunas of mind, body, and spirit in balance and maintain equilibrium so that the practitioner can reach the higher self, seeing and knowing the truth without the false distractions of one guna or another.

CLASSICAL YOGA: PATAÑJALI

Classical yoga of *Patañjali*, written down around the second century AD in the treatise known as the *Yoga Sutra*, was the first systemization of yoga. It is based on the Samkhya philosophy of creation and consciousness but goes a step further.

Where Samkhya taught that spiritual knowledge is all that is necessary to attain final liberation, Patañjali asserts that no one gets there through study alone. It takes hard work, in the form of ascetic practices and austere meditation, to ascend to a higher level of consciousness or cosmic understanding.

This work was not only mental but physical as well. Just because the work was difficult, however, did not mean the yogin should get agitated or strive to complete a goal at any cost. Yoga exercises were never about satisfying particular ambitions, but stemmed from a calm desire to pass over the human predicament and onto a higher plane.

This yoga also differed from Samkhya by introducing a god into the mix. Isvara was not a creator-god but rather an entity that existed for all eternity without being caught up in the illusion of being part of Nature. Like the sound of *Om,* Isvara acted as a vehicle to aid meditation and help the yogin attain liberation.

The goal in Patañjali's *Yoga Sutra* is for the yogin to suppress his or her mental states or activity (*citta*) through a series of physical exercises and breath control designed to conquer all mental activity and physical desire. These mental states produce a series of fluctuations (*vrittis*) that impede the yogin's ability to transcend human suffering. As soon as the yogin understands that the cittavritti binds him to the pain of the human condition, the cittavritti can be suppressed. However, to prevent its inevitable return, a strong and continual discipline is required. Only through the rigors of yoga, says Patañjali, can a person break this "circuit of psychic matter" and stop repeating painful actions.

The goal of yoga, therefore, is to stop the flow of cittavritti, or mental fluctuations. In other words, a yogin strives not to think and to stop random thoughts, sensations, memories, and words coming at him from external stimuli, as well as from his subconscious. The second thing a yogin attempts to quiet is the activity of his subconscious. According to yoga philosophy, the activity in the subconscious is responsible for propelling one's consciousness into action.

To help stop the flow of cittavritti, the yogin learns to concentrate on a single point or object. This object can be imaginary or concrete: a point between the eyebrows, a statue or painting, a mantra, a thought, or a color. This one-pointed concentration, called *ekagrata,* prevents the yogin from allowing his mind to attach itself to every object or thought that comes along. Ekagrata is not easy to achieve. If the body, for example, is tired or unhealthy, ekagrata is impossible to attain. Patañjali outlined a series of techniques designed to prepare the yogin for ekagrata and ultimately for final liberation. These stages include:

- *yamas* (restraints or moral observances)
- *niyamas* (disciplines or practices)
- *asanas* (postures or poses)
- *pranayama* (breath control)
- *pratyahara* (withdrawal or sensory inhibition)
- *dharana* (concentration)
- *dhyana* (meditation)
- *samadhi* (final liberation)

The first two groups—the yamas and niyamas—are the preparatory exercises that every yogin must adhere to before he or she is ready to embark on the yogic path.

Yamas. Sanskrit for "restraints," the yamas are the yogic equivalents of the Ten Commandments and serve as the foundation of all spiritual discipline. Patañjali defines five yamas as follows:

Nonviolence means that the yogin will abstain from harming anyone in any way, through words or actions. Nonviolence became associated with the spread of vegetarianism and nonviolent protests in India. Mahatma Gandhi was the most famous example of someone who practiced nonviolence both personally and in his political life. According to Patañjali, it was the great vow that should pervade all other actions.

Truthfulness means that one should never speak with the intent of harming, deceiving, or confusing another. According to the *Yoga Sutra*, a yogin should speak only to impart the truth and to share his or her knowledge with others.

Nonstealing not only means to refrain from taking anything that doesn't belong to you, but to refrain from coveting someone else's property, even in his thoughts.

Sexual continence, or chastity, is another key. Any yogin who forswears sexual intercourse (even thoughts of a sexual nature) gains vital energy. A later text, the *Agni-Purana*, defines it as the "renunciation of the eight degrees of sexual activity": fantasizing, glorifying the sex act, foreplay, eyeing the opposite sex, love talk, longing, deciding to break one's vow of chastity, and making love.

Nongreed came to mean in later texts giving up all your worldly possessions, but in the *Yoga Sutra* it meant one should only keep what's necessary and, more important, not become attached to the possessions. Patañjali taught that strict adherence to nongreed awarded the yogin knowledge of his past lives. Other texts list as many as ten yamas, which include sympathy, patience, steadfastness, proper diet, living in solitude, cleanliness, devotion to the guru, moral integrity, and dispassion.

Niyamas. The second limb of Patañjali's eightfold path, niyamas are disciplines. Like the yamas, the niyamas constitute five practices.

Purity, or cleanliness, taken to an extreme may lead to a repulsion toward the body—one's own and other people's. In the *Yoga Sutra*, cleansing the body meant both external and internal purification rituals. The external rituals included washing the body with water and sometimes with mud or earth; eating foods that promote lightness, clarity, strength, and happiness; and purifying the organs to eliminate toxins and alimentary residues. Internal cleansing meant paying attention to one's mental impurities, too. These purification rituals took on a larger role in the later Tantric practices of Hatha yoga.

Contentment, or serenity, is defined by Patañjali as the "absence of the desire to increase life's necessities," and says that perfecting it brings "unexcelled joy."

Asceticism has had several interpretations. Whereas some yogic traditions revile the body and define asceticism as allowing the body's desiccation, or emaciation, Patañjali's definition is more positive, teaching that asceticism leads to "perfection of the body and the senses." It leads to the transcendence of opposites or extremes and the control over oneself. A yogin who perfects the discipline of asceticism feels neither heat nor cold; the desire to sit is the same as the desire to stand; and the desire to speak is kept to a minimum lest the yogin reveal the inner secrets of the mind.

Study is not just book learning or memorization. It constitutes learning from one's guru the sacred knowledge needed for self-understanding and liberation. It also includes reciting the mantra *Om*.

Devotion to Isvara (God) means that the yogin desires to make God the object of all his or her actions. In exchange, Isvara bestows on the yogin a special love that aids him or her in practice. Many other niyamas show up in later yogic texts. Some of these include modesty, conviction, hospitality, fasting, bathing, silence, control of the penis, and following the teacher's footsteps; the more devotional disciplines include worship, pilgrimages, affirmation of the existence of the divine, and adoration in their niyamas.

Asanas. Once the student begins the practices of restraint and discipline in earnest, the real yoga techniques can begin. Asana in the *Yoga Sutra* of Patañjali refers to postures designed to give the body stability and strength and to help establish control of the physical body. Patañjali doesn't go into much detail about such postures except to say that the yogin should be able to hold the body in a particular position for long periods of time without effort. It's only when one no longer feels fatigue or pain in certain areas of the body that one can give up paying any attention to the body itself and devote oneself completely to meditation, or ekagrata.

Pranayama. After a yogin has begun to perfect his asana practice, he is ready to conquer the breath. Pranayama (literally meaning "breath extension") in the *Yoga Sutra* prolongs life itself and rejuvenates the body. The goal in practicing pranayama is to calm the breath and make its rhythm as slow as possible. By concentrating on controlling the movement of the breath (retaining the breath between the inhalation and the exhalation—inhale, hold; exhale, hold), the yogin slows and ultimately steadies the movement of the mind and the senses. The first step in learning pranayama is to perfect the three phases of breathing: inhalation, retention, and exhalation. More advanced yogins can retain the breath at will. Later yoga schools (Tantric and Hatha) believed that practicing proper pranayama techniques cured a multitude of physical ailments.

Pratyahara. This fifth stage of Patañjali's eightfold yogic path is the beginning of the path that tames the senses and the mind. The first four stages on the eightfold path prepare the yogin for the rigors of this and the next three stages. Literally meaning "withdrawal," pratyahara enables the yogin to separate his or her senses from the tangible world. This means that yogins make a conscious effort to draw their senses and attention away from the external world and become less distracted by outside stimuli. They remain keenly aware of all the senses but cultivate a feeling of detachment at the same time. Directing attention inward, yogins quiet the mind and begin to observe their minds and bodies more objectively. It's a time for them to take a look at habits that may not only be detrimental to their physical health but their spiritual pursuit, too.

Dharana. The practice of pratyahara helps the yogin to prepare for dharana, or intense concentration. The yogin has now learned to rid him- or herself of all outside distractions. Now he or she must train the mind to rid itself of all scattered thoughts. Practicing asana and pranayama helped the yogin pay attention, first to the body and then to the breath. Pratyahara helped slow activity even more, and the yogin became more focused. Now dharana allows the yogin to concentrate on a single point, that is, to practice ekagrata. As we learned earlier, that focal point can be anything: the navel, the space between the eyebrows, a flower, an image of a guru, Isvara, or a sound or phrase (mantra).

Dhyana. The ability to concentrate on a single point prepares the yogin for the next two stages. Dhyana is the uninterrupted flow of concentration, a deepening of dharana. Patañjali allows the yogin to use any object as a prop for meditation, as long as it isn't taboo or doesn't arouse the yogin. Although Patañjali allows the yogin to use props, such as diagrams or images of Sanskrit symbols, the goal of dhyana should be complete quieting of the mind.

Samadhi. During samadhi, or ultimate liberation, the yogin becomes one with the point of focus and transcends the self altogether. Union of opposites becomes possible—life is no different from death, emptiness equals abundance, subject and object merge, and being and nonbeing are the same thing.

This is a very hard concept to understand, especially for the Western mind. Basically, the yogin realizes that all entities are interconnected and the individual self returns to its primordial place in the higher self. Another way of explaining it is that the yogin understands there is no separation between the one meditating and the object of the meditation. Also the yogin is no longer troubled by external tensions and is impervious to hot and cold, light and darkness; he becomes stronger and more self-contained and able to protect himself from any outside stimuli. Consciousness becomes absorbed, and the spirit is in a state of truth and bliss.

POSTCLASSICAL YOGA

The postclassical period of yoga begins around the second century AD. During this time, yoga changed dramatically. The *Yoga-Upanishads*, one of the later Upanishads, describe the techniques of yoga, adhering pretty much to Patañjali's eightfold path: restraints, disciplines, postures, breath control, sensory withdrawal, concentration, meditation, and liberation. But they go further and are more sophisticated than Patañjali.

Most of them mention particular postures (asanas) by name; they define different schools of yoga: Mantra yoga, Laya yoga, Raja yoga, and Hatha yoga; they talk more about breathing techniques; and they glorify yogic abilities. The *Yoga-Upanishads* discuss physiology in great detail and explain how the macrocosm (the universe) is inherent in the microcosm (the body). It is during this period of yogic development that the overall health of the yogin becomes an important prerequisite to attaining enlightenment.

Mantra yoga is a relatively late development of yoga. Reciting various mantras made up of sounds or syllables from the Sanskrit alphabet enables the yogin to attain liberation. We know from the *Rgveda* that mantras have long been invoked for their magical powers and as a means to perfect sacrificial rituals. Mantra yoga is said to be good for beginning yoga students.

Helpful for the intermediate student, Laya yoga uses hand gestures, pranayama, and meditation on the body (particularly the immortality of the body) to attain physical and psychological control, longevity, and ultimately liberation. Its goal is to dissolve the individual ego, or conditional mind, and absorb it into the Absolute.

Raja yoga is the so-called royal yoga outlined in Patañjali's *Yoga Sutra*. In the later *Yoga-Upanishads*, Raja yoga was compared to Hatha yoga, which was merely the means of preparing the body for the higher spiritual practices of Raja yoga.

TANTRIC YOGA

By the middle of the fourth century AD, Tantric yoga became incredibly popular. With its emphasis on the physical body, Tantra was a departure from the classical and postclassical schools of yogic meditation. Tantric philosophy was not new, however; many scholars believe its roots date back to the practices of the early Brahmanic people or even the Indus Valley culture.

Like in most yogic traditions, Tantra teaches that primordial consciousness contains within itself all sets of opposites. Humanity is caught up in the illusion of opposites. The goal of the tantrika (one who practices Tantra), then, is to reunite the opposing principles in one's own body.

Before a practitioner can delve into practices to attain liberation, he or she must be well-versed in the yamas and niyamas, as well as the poses and breathing practices we learned about from Patañjali's eightfold yogic path. The first place to begin for a practitioner is with concentration and meditation on an icon of a deity. Although this seems easy enough, it isn't; it requires intense, uninterrupted concentration and a summoning of spiritual energies.

After the practitioner perfects the ability to meditate on an icon, the next step is visualization. This allows the student not only to see and feel the sacred force of the deity as a mental exercise but to experience its divinity. When the student is ready, he incorporates the deity into particular parts of his body in ritual projection. For example, associating the five fingers of one's hand with the five gross elements (ether, air, fire, water, and earth).

Mantras—mystical sounds—take on a whole new meaning in Tantra. Imparted only by a guru, mantras assist the practitioner in his meditation. A mantra is generally just a syllable or a string of syllables and may not have any translatable meaning. The use of mantra is very ritualistic. It's not enough in Tantra simply to recite the mantra in one's meditation. One must purify one's thoughts first, be alert and physically strong, and begin to dissect the mantra, letter by letter. Invoking a mantra awakens the corresponding parts of the body and the forces of the universe it represents.

Mandalas are used to help the yogin become one with his deity. Mandalas are drawings on wood, cloth, or paper—sometimes simple, other times quite complex—of circles and geometric elements. In the center of all mandalas resides the "seed" that represents the point of true realization, the union of the cosmos and the mind. Surrounding circles depict all the levels of existence. The mandala represents the outside world and the cosmos; by entering the mandala through meditation and visualization, the yogin enters sacred space and sees the gods residing in his own heart. He understands there is no separation between the individual and the Absolute.

HATHA YOGA

In yoga, health and physical conditioning have always been a means of controlling the body to discipline the mind. While the body and mind were seen as microcosms of the universe even in Vedic times, most yogins disdained the body, seeing it as the source of great pain and a hindrance to their goal of final liberation. Other yogins understood the necessity of keeping a strong, healthy body to enable them to withstand the pressures of meditation practice. Patañjali, while acknowledging the importance of the physical body, believed that the purer a yogin's consciousness became, the more the yogin viewed the body as defiled and the more he shunned others for fear of becoming contaminated by their physical presence.

The popularization of Tantra changed all that. Its practitioners revered the physical body and saw it as a means of conquering death. Tantra taught that one attained liberation through experiencing life to the fullest. But of all the schools of thought in yoga, Hatha yoga was the one that focused on physicalness the most.

Hatha taught a systematic approach to mastering the body: One must learn the complete physiology (organs, energy channels, tissues, and the presiding divinities) to transform the physical body into the subtle, divine body and thereby attain liberation. As in Tantra, sexual practices also come into play in the Hatha yoga texts as a means of unifying the male and female energies. But in general, Hatha yoga is associated with strenuous physical postures as opposed to the sex of the Tantra. There are not many texts remaining from the Hatha yoga school of thought. Of those that do exist, only three shed any light on its practices. The earliest one, the *Hathayogapradipika*, describes approximately 15 postures (asanas), most of them variations of the lotus position. The *Hathayogapradipika* includes techniques to:

- purify the body and bring it into balance
- control and extend the breath
- increase digestion
- aid concentration

The second text is the *Gheranda Samhita*, which describes 32 different postures and 25 seals (mudras). The sage Gheranda focused on purification rituals called *shodhanas*, part of his sevenfold discipline of yoga. The third treatise, the *Shiva Samhita*, is the most extensive. It gives us an elaborate breakdown of yogic physiology and describes five different types of prana, or life breath, and how to regulate them through pranayama, asanas, and mudras. Eighty-four different asanas are mentioned, but the *Samhita* gives detailed accounts of only four of them. The physical postures are touted for their ability to cure diseases, bestow longevity, and confer magical powers.

Before a yogin can even begin the physical practice of Hatha yoga, he or she must purify the body. The following are six techniques his guru would employ.

Dhautis. These purification rites concentrate on internal cleansing, dental cleansing, rectal cleansing, and purifying the heart.

Internal cleansing practices range from simple techniques, such as belching or passing gas; to more challenging ones, such as pushing the navel back toward the spine 100 times to stimulate the digestive fires in the belly; to rather severe ones, such as washing one's prolapsed intestines—not something one would want to do unsupervised! Dental cleansing involves brushing the teeth, the tongue, the ears, and the sinuses. Cleaning the ears promotes the ability to hear inner sounds. Rectal cleansing by means of a turmeric stalk helps the breath to circulate freely. Cleansing the heart is an intense practice. The first part includes taking a stalk of turmeric, placing it down one's gullet, and slowly drawing it out. This helps remove excess pitta (bile) and kapha (phlegm) from the mouth and chest. The second technique is "cleansing by vomiting," a way of removing kapha from the stomach and chest, which comprises eating a full meal, drinking water until it fills up to the throat, gazing up between the eyebrows, and throwing up the water. The third part is the most difficult to perform: Swallow a long, thick piece of cloth and leave it in the stomach for a while before pulling it out again. This is said to help reduce fever and cure diseases of the stomach and large intestine, leprosy, and other skin disorders.

Bastis. The bastis are nothing but enemas—dry or water-based. The dry enema works in the seated, forward-bent position, contracting and dilating the sphincter muscle and pressing down hard on the intestines. The water enema also calls on the yogin to contract and dilate the sphincter muscle, but this time he or she squats in water up to the navel in the chair pose. This is said to cure urinary and digestive troubles.

Netis. The netis clear out the nasal passages and the sinuses. These days people use a neti pot to pour salted water in one nostril and allow it to drain out the other side. Another method works by inserting thin threads into the nostrils and pulling them out through the mouth. This is said to improve vision and clear the sinus cavities.

Nauli. The nauli is actually a yoga pose designed to balance the digestive system. To perform nauli, sit in the lotus pose, bend forward slightly, and release the shoulders forward (hollowing out the chest). Isolate the *rectus abdominis* muscle (the large, straight muscle in the abdomen), lock it in place, and then rotate it vigorously for several minutes.

Trataka. Trataka is designed to cure diseases of the eye and to encourage clairvoyance. It involves sitting in the lotus pose and staring at a small object directly in front of one's feet. One should stare at the object, without blinking, until one's eyes begin to tear uncontrollably.

Kapala Bhati. The sixth cleansing act is usually made up of three practices. In the first, or left process, the yogin inhales repeatedly through the left nostril and exhales through the right. In the second, the yogin draws water up through the nose and expels it through the mouth. The third technique works the opposite way: The yogin draws water into the mouth, holds his breath for as long as possible, and expels the water through the nose, making the sound "sheet" as he exhales. This practice claims to control hunger, thirst, and sleep.

HATHA YOGIC PHYSIOLOGY

In Ayurvedic medicine and perhaps as far back as the Vedic period, physicians understood something about basic anatomy. No doubt most yogic gurus were also well-versed in scientific physiology, but for purposes of meditation and to awaken "primordial consciousness," the yogins used a more spiritual or mystical physiologic model. Instead of talking about muscles, veins, nerves, and organs the way a medical scientist would, a yogin would expound on the theory of the nadis, the chakras, the physical body, and the subtle body.

Just like Ayurvedic practitioners, Hatha yogins viewed the body as a microcosm of the universe. They all saw the five elements—ether, air, fire, water, and earth—absorbed in the body. For example, the cosmic winds (*vayu*) are incorporated into the body as air or breath (*vata*); fire (*agni*) becomes the digestive fire. In Hatha yoga, the spinal column is a miniature Mount Meru—the mountain at the center of the Earth. Therefore, the spinal column is seen as the central axis of the body that controls everything. Yogins see this axis as one large bone that is fixed and motionless. The seven worlds of Hindu cosmology are represented in the seven chakras, or psychoenergetic centers, in the body.

The central axis of the body is just one of a multitude of veins, arteries, and nerves present in the body. Yogic texts differ on the number of these channels, or nadis, that help transport the life force (*prana*), which flows through the physical body. Estimations vary from 10 to 700 million of these vessels. The three most important of these are the *sushumna*, the *ida*, and the *pingala*.

The ida nadi, also called the "channel of comfort," is responsible for cooling the body and encouraging it to exhale. It moves the down-breath of the body during the exhalation or during suspension of the breath at the bottom of the exhale. The ida nadi is said to begin just above the sex organs and terminate under the left nostril. It controls the lower half of the body, from the navel down to the feet.

The pingala nadi's nature is strong, expansive, and energizing, encouraging the yogin to inhale. This nadi moves the life force through the body, on the inhalation or during breath retention at the top of the inhalation, creating heat and light and invigorating the whole person. A clear pingala nadi optimizes respiration and cardiovascular functioning.

The sushumna nadi is, for the physical body, the central axis (or spinal column), which transports the life force from the base of the spine up to the crown of the head. Inside the sushumna is a thinner, finer channel; and inside that is a channel as thin as one-thousandth of a hair width, where the chakras are said to attach.

All humans contain within them a multitude of nadis that transport the vital energy to all parts of the body. It's important to keep these channels of transportation pure and unobstructed, otherwise illness occurs. The most common and effective purification practices are called *nirmanu* and *samanu*. Nirmanu is the same as the dhauti practices discussed earlier: cleaning the teeth, the gastrointestinal tract, the nasal passages, and the heart. The samanu practice involves breathing practice, which a yogin performs while seated in the lotus pose. During the exercise, the yogin must visualize his or her guru, bringing the teacher into his or her heart. It begins by meditating on the syllable *yam* (symbol of the cosmic wind).

- First inhale through the left nostril while silently chanting *yam* 16 times.
- Hold the breath while silently chanting *yam* 64 times.
- Exhale very slowly (32 repetitions of *yam*) through the right nostril.
- Concentrate on the fire in the belly, drawing it up to the heart.
- Inhale through the right nostril while silently chanting *ram* (the fire syllable) 16 times.
- Retain the breath while silently chanting *ram* 64 times.
- Exhale very slowly (32 repetitions of *ram*).
- Meditate on the reflection of the moon—the nectar of immortality—at the tip of the nose.
- Repeat inhalation on the left side using the syllable *tham;* retain the breath for 64 counts while meditating on the immortal nectar; and then exhale for 32 counts, silently chanting to oneself the syllable *lam.*
- Perform the adept's posture—similar to the lotus pose but with the left heal against the anus and the right one above the genitals. Rest the chin on the chest and gaze at a point right between the eyebrows.

Deep within the sushumna channel lie the *chakras*: psychoenergetic centers where the subtle body meets the physical body. These centers house all the energy necessary for a human to live, and they distribute that energy through the thousands of nadis. Most texts agree that there are seven main chakras, including the sahasrara chakra, which resides above the crown of the head and transcends all physical existence.

The chakras are a type of internal map that a yogin uses as he or she meditates on the body. The yogin meditates on each chakra as a lotus blossom with a certain number of petals, each with a Sanskrit letter imprinted on it. Each chakra has a corresponding color, a ruling god or goddess, and a "seed syllable" from the Sanskrit alphabet. Each chakra also relates to one of the five gross elements.

Beginning with the base of the spine, the seven major chakras are as follows:

Muladhara chakra—this root chakra resides at the base of the spine. Its element is earth; its sense is the sense of smell; its organ of action is the feet; and its sound is *lam*. This chakra is the source of desire, and Dakini is the goddess that presides over it.

Svadishthana chakra—Situated in the genital area, this is also known as the pleasant chakra. Its element is water; its sense is taste; its organ of action is the hands; and its sound is *vam*.

Manipura chakra—This chakra sits right in the lumbar region of the spine, at the level of the navel. Its element is fire; its sense is sight; its organ of action is the gastrointestinal tract; and its sound is *ram*. It governs the breath and the emotions of fear, jealousy, and shame. To contemplate this chakra successfully is said to bring the yogin freedom from disease and pain and the ability to make medicinal remedies.

Anahata chakra—Located at the heart, this chakra has been known as a powerful center of the body since Vedic times. Its element is air; its sense is touch; the organ of action is the penis; and its sound is *yam*. It is the seat of the individual self. Isvara resides here. It governs emotions such as hope, anxiety, doubt, remorse, duty, and egotism.

Vishuddha chakra—This is the throat chakra, whose color is gold. Its element is ether, or space; its sense is hearing; its organ of action is the mouth; and its sound is *ham*.

Ajña chakra—Situated between the eyebrows, this chakra governs the realm of understanding and the power of concentration. It is sometimes known as the third eye. It has no element; its sense is the sense of cognition; its organ of action is yoni, or female genitalia, and its sound is *Om*.

Sahasrara chakra—Beyond the crown of the head sits the "Lotus of One Thousand Petals," the place of transcendence. The sahasrara chakra represents pure consciousness. It encompasses all colors, all sounds, all organs of action, all functions of the mind and body. It symbolizes the final union of Shiva (male) and Shakti (female).

KUNDALINI—YOGIC UNION

Tantra and Hatha yoga took two basic, ancient principles of Indian philosophy—Samkhya philosophy and the body as a microcosm of the universe—and expanded upon them. In Samkhya, Cosmic Consciousness (Purusha) was masculine, formless, immobile, and omniscient Matter, and Nature (Prakriti) was feminine, creative, and the ever-moving Spirit. In yoga, the god Shiva personifies the Purusha, and the goddess Shakti is the feminine form, Prakriti. The union of these two aspects of the Divine represents the reunion of all opposites and the liberation from the cycle of birth, death, and rebirth.

Viewing the body as a microcosm of the divine dance, Tantra and Hatha yoga saw the Shiva and Shakti residing in all of us. Kundalini yoga saw that the path to uniting these opposites was to combine sexuality and spirit in the human form. The union of Shiva and Shakti awakens the yogin, destroying any sense of the individual self and flooding his or her entire being with indescribable bliss. To prepare the body and mind for this union, the yogin must practice asanas, pranayama, selected mudras, and bandhas (locks). Though the primary goal of these practices is to release the flow of life force in the body, the asanas bring health benefits as well. Originally mentioned in Patañjali's *Yoga Sutra* as a way of sitting for meditation (the body should be steady, relaxed, and comfortable; the posture straight and in proper alignment), asana in Hatha yoga acquired a variety of therapeutic effects.

Pranayama became the principal way to awaken Kundalini energy and unite the higher consciousness for Hatha and Tantric yogins. Pranayama, when practiced properly, strengthens the body, invigorates the mind, and makes the practitioner feel younger. Pranayama's purpose is to expand the life force through inhalation, retention, and exhalation. Once the yogin is able to open the channels in his body (the ida, pingala, and sushumna nadis) to allow for the unimpeded flow of energy, he is ready to learn to control where the energy goes. There are two ways to do this: through the practice of mudras, or seals, and by creating bandhas, or locks, which prevent the energy from entering a particular chakra or area in the body.

Paramudras are practices that combine asana, pranayama, bandhas, and mudras—are highly esoteric practices, the details of which have never been written down. It has been claimed that these can only be transmitted orally and performed under the supervision of an experienced guru. A sampling of paramudras are as follows:

Mahamudra (the Great Seal)—The yogin sits with the right leg outstretched and the left foot pressing against the perineum, holding the right foot with his hands. He then closes off all orifices of the body (ears, eyes, nose, and mouth) using his powers of concentration, and contracts the throat by placing his chin on his chest snugly while gazing between the eyebrows and retaining the breath. This activates all the nadis and stops the flow of semen, which increases vitality. Modern yogins believe this paramudra relieves constipation, hemorrhoids, and indigestion.

Khecharimudra (the air-moving seal)—There's some preparation involved before the yogin can perform khecharimudra. He first must cut the tongue's frenum (the connecting membrane that keeps the tongue in place), and massage the tongue with milk, stretching it out (sometimes using an iron tool) until it is long enough to reach a point between the eyebrows. Then the yogin must loosen his soft palate by hooking a piece of metal onto the palate ridge and gently drawing it forward. After he is ready (and the procedure could take several months), the yogin draws his tongue back down his gullet, blocking the nasal passages that open into the mouth, silently repeats the mantras his guru has given him, and fixes his gaze between his eyebrows. This supposedly blocks the flow of semen; prevents fainting, hunger, thirst, old age, and death; and makes the yogin immune to snakebites.

Vajrolimudra (the thunderbolt seal)—This practice is said to enable the yogin to combine (in his own body) the male and female fluids, thereby uniting all opposites. Months of preparation are necessary for this one, too. The man must cleanse and strengthen his penis, making it as strong and hard as a thunderbolt. He then practices dipping it into a bronze vessel of cow's milk, sucking the milk up with his penile shaft, and releasing it again. The bandha he perfects is called the *medhra bandha,* or phallus lock, by which he causes the penis to stay rigid for an indefinite period of time. When he is ready, he ejaculates his semen into a woman's vagina where it mixes with her fluid. He then sucks the two fluids back up into his body. This mudra, not surprisingly, is said to be very deleterious to the female volunteer.

Other mudras and bandhas help the advanced practitioner to seal off the left and right channels (the pingala and the ida nadis), forcing all the Kundalini power to surge up through the sushumna nadi and head straight for the sahasrara chakra above the crown of the head.

YOGA AND WESTERN MEDICINE

Yoga came to America with the arrival of Swami Vivekananda. It wasn't the physical style of Hatha yoga that so intrigued the participants that day at the World Parliament of Religions, but it was the merits of Patañjali's ancient eightfold path of practice. It took many years for the practice to catch on, and it took many years after that for its health benefits to be noticed by the medical establishment.

Yoga, for millennia, has taught that the body, mind, and breath are inexorably linked. Yogins discovered as they worked to attain liberation, one side benefit they produced was a physically fit, healthy body free of the normal aches, pains, and afflictions. Modern Western medicine saw this side effect as one of primary importance to a people whose lives are filled with stress, poor eating habits, and little time to exercise. Besides toning and strengthening, yoga benefits all the systems of the body: muscular, skeletal, circulatory, respiratory, digestive, reproductive, endocrine, lymphatic, and nervous. The combination of posture, movement, and breath also affects the emotions and the mind. Actions, knowledge, and spirit form a harmonic trinity. Mainstream medical practitioners and researchers have begun to take a serious look at the benefits of yoga. They have found that heart patients who stick to a combined regimen of yoga, meditation, and a low-fat diet can reverse coronary artery blockage. Combinations of yoga and other meditation have been shown to help patients manage stress and chronic pain and even reduce blood pressure.

Yoga and yoga meditation help the practitioner not only manage stress better but to change the stress-producing patterns the mind sets up. They remove the obstacles—the causes—of the stress and discomfort, and they help the practitioner develop a deeper insight into what causes agitation in the first place.

BENEFITS OF ASANAS

Several asanas also work to balance the body and mind:

Padmasana, the lotus pose, is said to help overcome all manner of disease.

Muktasana involves a similar seated pose in which the left ankle sits above the groin and the right ankle above that.

Vajrasana is a pose in which the yogin grips the thighs "like a thunderbolt," and places his or her legs underneath the anus. It works to strengthen the body.

Bhujangasana is known today as cobra pose. Lying on the stomach and pressing up through the arms, the yogin lifts the body from the navel up, arching the back and raising the head like a snake. The cobra pose is said to increase body temperature, cure myriad diseases, and awaken the Kundalini or "serpent" energy.

Mritasana, or corpse pose, involves lying supine on the ground, completely relaxed, to overcome fatigue and regenerate energy after practicing asanas.

Some of the other benefits that modern Western medicine has begun to recognize in yoga are:

- increased immune system functioning
- increased musculoskeletal flexibility (aiding in the treatment and prevention of arthritis, multiple sclerosis, scoliosis, fibromyalgia, and injuries)
- decreased discomfort in premenstrual syndrome and menopause
- enhanced mood and stability in mental illnesses such as depression

JAPAN

The ancient healing traditions of Japan are closely connected to those of China. Starting in the sixth century AD, an extensive cultural exchange existed between Japan and China. Ideas about medicine, religion, philosophy, and even the method of writing were transmitted to Japan by the Chinese. Therefore, much of the traditional medicine practiced in Japan relies heavily on traditional Chinese theory and technique.

Before this period of interaction with China, however, Japan's history is somewhat shrouded. Our understanding of medical practices and beliefs before that time is based on records of ancient tales and legends that were not systematically compiled until the eighth century AD, and even these are of questionable reliability. Japan is also unique in relation to other countries in Asia in that it adopted western European medicine and made it a matter of national policy in the mid-1800s. In doing so, Japan deliberately relegated the medical traditions that it had relied on for centuries to second-class status.

PRACTICES IN PREHISTORY

The origin of the Japanese people continues to be debated. One perspective is that two successive waves of peoples came to settle the islands. One wave from northern Asia is associated with the Jomon period (2000–200 BC) and another group of peoples from southeast Asia is associated with the Yayoi period (200 BC–AD 200). Little is known about the most ancient medical traditions in the periods preceding the sixth century AD. Since writing first arrived in Japan from China in the sixth century and was not routinely used by the Japanese until the seventh century, many of the descriptions of ancient practices had only been transmitted orally.

The compilations of ancient histories, tales, and legends—known as the *Nihongi* and the *Kojiki*—and accounts of early life in Japan—the *Fudoki*—describe some of the beliefs and practices of the early Japanese people, at least as they were understood in the early part of the eighth century.

According to the *Nihongi*, two divine beings—Opo-kuni-nushi and Su-kanabiko-no-mikoto—joined their powers to build the universe. These two beings "also determined the method of curing illnesses for the race of mortal man and for animals; they also determined magical methods for doing away with calamities from birds, beasts, and creeping things."

SHINTO

Shinto (or *Kami-No-Michi*, meaning "the way of the gods") was the name given to the indigenous religious traditions of Japan. Shinto was not that significant in the development of traditional medicine in Japan, but it was important to popular ideas associated with healing, such as bathing practices and spiritual interventions for disease. Japan has a long history of incorporating the advances and practices of other cultures into its own—in medicine, it was no different. When the more medically significant Buddhist practices arrived in Japan, they intermingled with Shinto and were often used simultaneously or interchangeably, eventually leading to distinctive adaptations of Chinese practices.

Ancient tales describe the use of native plants to treat disease, sometimes in a magical context. One tale that is often referred to and was recorded in the *Kojiki* describes the instructions given by a divine being, or *Kami*, to a rabbit who had lost his fur in an unhappy encounter with a crocodile. The rabbit is sent to the river to bathe his body with water and then to roll in the pollen of the *kama* grass that grows at the mouth of the river. Throughout the centuries, similar plants such as kudzu would be used both in the folk traditions of herbal medicine in Japan and in the formal herbal traditions imported from China.

RITUALS OF CLEANSING

The early Japanese view of the world made no clear distinction between gods and men. Human beings were seen as essentially good, but transgressions and misdeeds could allow evil spirits to cause disease and calamities. The misdeeds and, hence, the illness could be remedied through rituals of purification.

Purification had other uses as well. Contact with polluted people or things, such as blood, corpses, and people with skin diseases, could produce the condition of "having a spirit polluted by bad poison." The ideas of physical injury and uncleanliness were closely linked; the expression *kega*, for example, has the meaning of both a "wound" and a "defilement." As a result, association with the ill, the dead, and the dying was potentially very problematic—a belief not conducive to recruiting medical practitioners. However, contact with defiling objects, people, or situations could be counteracted by cleansing rituals such as bathing the body and rinsing the mouth. Ancient ideas of illness included the notion of contact with, or even penetration by, the unclean, which would have to be removed forcefully and definitively. Consequently, medicines that produced sweating, purgation, and vomiting were popular. The idea of certain situations and contacts as dangerously impure continue to be prevalent in contemporary Japan, although in less extreme forms.

CHINESE MEDICINE COMES TO JAPAN

The ancient medical traditions of Japan are so closely linked with Chinese medicine, it is typical for many discussions of traditional medicine in Japan actually to begin with a description of traditional medicine in China. Kon Mu is said to be the first physician to come to Japan using Chinese methods. He was sent in AD 414 by the king of Silla, in southeast Korea, to treat the emperor Inkyo Tenno. It is quite possible, though, that there was some degree of medical exchange prior to this date, because there is evidence of some interaction between the people of the Japanese islands and the people of the mainland from about AD 57.

In 562, Zhi Chong (*Chiso* in Japanese) came from southern China with more than 100 books on the practice of Chinese medicine, including the *Systematic Classic of Acupuncture* (*Zhen Jiu Jia Yi Jing*) and probably the *Classic of Difficulties* (*Nan Jing*). These exchanges coincide with the adoption of Chinese characters as the basis for Japanese writing and the gradual expansion of literacy throughout the elite of Japanese society. With the establishment of direct contact between Japan and China in the sixth century, Japanese physicians traveled to China to learn more about its healing traditions. The movement of information was no longer in the form of texts and a few physicians arriving from China or Korea. By 608, young Japanese physicians began to travel to China for long periods to study these medical texts and examine patients with Chinese physicians.

Medicine was not the only thing Japan appropriated from China. In the early centuries of the exchange, Japan made an effort to model its social organization and imperial administration on China's. One effort to emulate the bureaucratic structures of China was the creation of the Taiho Code in 702. This code made provision for a ministry of health to be composed of specialists, physicians, students, and researchers. The Chinese model proved to be difficult for the Japanese, not because of the science, but because of the different social and political natures of the two countries. One striking feature of China, for example, was the extensive use of examinations and other merit-based competitions to ensure that individuals achieved rank and authority based on competence. Because social rank was based on inherited position in Japan, the exam-based approach was not adopted. Also, the strong central authority of the emperor, which was an important factor in China's development, was not a feature of Japanese life. The emperor was of important symbolic value, but the power was held unequally by a number of feudal lords who did not fall under anything resembling central authority until the sixteenth century. Despite these challenges, Chinese medicine was well established in Japan by the early eighth century. Medical exchange continued during this period. One notable event involved the Chinese Buddhist monk Jian Zhen (*Kan Jin* in Japanese) from Yang Chow who moved to Japan in 753 along with

35 disciples, his medical books, and many herbs. Among these disciples were physicians who shared their medical knowledge with the Japanese monks and students. Jian Zhen is said to have created a charitable clinic where he and his disciples treated patients for free.

IMPORTANT MEDICAL BOOKS FROM CHINA

Between the sixth and ninth centuries, many important and famous medical texts arrived in Japan from China. These included books such as the *Yellow Emperor's Inner Classic* (*Huang Di Nei Jing*), which may have been compiled as early as 100 BC. The *Divine Husbandman's Classic of Materia Medica* (*Shen Nong Ben Cao*) appeared in Japan about this time as well. This text is the first known appearance of a formal presentation of medicinal substances considered individually. Working over the centuries, writers in both China and Japan would produce many texts describing the uses and properties of these and other medicinal substances.

The *Classic of Difficulties* (*Nan Jing*) was compiled sometime during the first or second century AD, although its authorship is attributed to the legendary physician Bian Que. This text has had, and continues to have, a marked influence on the practice of Chinese medicine and, to an even greater extent, on the practice of Chinese medicine in Japan. The *Classic of Difficulties* marks a drastic shift in medical thinking. It constitutes a systematic discussion of the theory and practice of therapeutic acupuncture. It is almost entirely devoid of magical elements. Because of its succinct and organized approach to therapy, this text retained its popularity in Japan in a way that it did not in China.

The *Treatise on Cold Damage* (*Shang Han Lun*) and the *Survey of Important Elements from the Golden Cabinet and Jade Container* (*Jin Gui Yao Lue*) were published in the second century AD by Zhang Zhong Jing (also known as Zhang Ji). Chinese medical texts of this period were primarily philosophical (except for the *Classic of Difficulties*), but Zhang studied disease more from a clinical standpoint, laying emphasis on the physical signs, symptoms, and course of disease, as well as the method of treatment. (He was especially interested in fevers because most of his village was wiped out by fever epidemics, possibly typhoid.) The Treatise on Cold Damage became, perhaps, the single most influential text on the practice of herbal medicine in Japan. It came to function as the core text of herbal medicine, or *kanpo* (Chinese method), in Japan. Zhang's book was theoretically and diagnostically sophisticated, but its emphasis on therapy rather than theory made it popular with practical-minded Japanese physicians. The *Treatise on Cold Damage* inspired many commentaries and an entire school of medical thought in the seventeenth century. Today many of its formulas are approved for insurance reimbursement by the Japanese government.

FUNDAMENTAL CONCEPTS

With some slight variations, most of the theory underlying traditional Japanese medicine is the same as traditional Chinese medicine. Yin and yang, the five phases, and *ki* (the Japanese version of the Chinese *qi*) came to be the important organizing principles just as they did in China.

YIN AND YANG

Yin and yang express the idea of opposing but complementary phenomena that exist in a state of dynamic equilibrium. The most ancient expression of this idea seems to have been that of the shady and sunny sides of a hill. The sunlit southern side was the yang side and the shaded or northern side was the yin side. The contrast between the bright and dark sides of the hill portrayed the yang and the yin. Yin and yang are always present simultaneously; there is no absolute yin or absolute yang. There is no yin without yang; something is yin only in relation to something else being yang and vice versa.

The *Yellow Emperor's Inner Classic*, the oldest text to discuss the medical application of yin and yang, tells us that "yin and yang are the way of heaven and earth." This text used yin and yang to express ideas about normal physiology and disease processes as well.

Yin and yang were applied to the organization of phenomena in many ways. The ideas and properties associated with yin and yang are often illustrated with lists of associated terms. Yang, for example, is considered to be hot and rapid and to move upward. Yin is cold and slow, and it moves downward. These contrasts allow the physician to organize his thought about the body in a systematic way. Thus, a yin or cold condition such as arthritis would be treated with yang or warm therapies such as moxibustion and warming herbs.

THE FIVE PHASES

Another idea that has played a significant part in the development of some aspects of Chinese medicine is that of the five phases (*wu xing*): earth, metal, water, wood, and fire. The five phases are connected with all phenomena. Each phase has an associated taste, organ, emotion, food, and season. The relationships that exist between the phases also exist between the phenomena that are associated with them, and these ideas extend to diagnosis and therapy. For example, the kidneys, which are associated with water, are thought to nourish and support the liver, which is associated with wood according to the cycle of generation. Therefore, a problem with the kidneys might also go on to affect the liver.

The *Classic of Difficulties* made extensive use of the five-phase theory in the development of a system of pulse diagnosis that allowed the practitioner to diagnose disturbances in the channels and the organs and then use acupuncture to treat them. In ancient acupuncture traditions, each phase was said to relate to many different phenomena—everything from weather to seasons. By observing these relationships and understanding the interplay among the five elements, the ancient Japanese physician could understand the illnesses that afflicted his patients and prescribe the most effective treatments for them.

KI AND THE ESSENTIAL SUBSTANCES

Apart from the ideas of yin and yang and the five phases, there is no concept more crucial to Chinese medicine than *qi*. In Japanese, the character is pronounced *ki*. *Ki* is the subtle force that drives physiologic functions and maintains the health and vitality of the individual.

The idea of *ki* is extremely broad, encompassing almost every variety of natural, living phenomena. *Ki* was said to be produced as a result of normal physiologic processes and to circulate through *keiraku*, or channels. There are many different types of *ki* in the body, but in general, *ki* has the functions of activation, warming, defense, transformation, and containment.

DIAGNOSIS

A great deal has been said about diagnosis in the chapter on Chinese medicine. Traditionally in China, the idea of diagnosis included four methods: inspection, listening, palpation, and questioning. These ideas persist in Japanese therapeutic traditions, too. Over time, the Japanese medical tradition placed greater emphasis on palpation, or pulse diagnosis, than the Chinese, and sometimes, palpation alone was considered enough for a diagnosis.

It is interesting to note that at different times, certain practices were emphasized or de-emphasized in Japan. For example, some traditions of Japanese acupuncture entirely dispensed with pulse diagnosis in favor of palpating the abdomen, whereas others retained the pulse diagnosis as a key diagnostic tool.

THERAPEUTICS

Japanese approaches to therapy mirrored many Chinese practices and developed new ones. For example, acupuncture—the insertion of fine metal needles into the body to adjust the functioning of the channels and organs—was frequently used. Moxibustion—the burning of the plant moxa on or near certain points on the body—was also practiced.

Although originally similar treatments, these forms of therapy were elaborated on by the Japanese. The trends toward specialized development became so pronounced that by the twentieth century, the practices of acupuncture and moxibustion became separately licensed in Japan. This development has permitted the folk use of moxibustion by monks in Buddhist temples to persist.

In the middle part of this century, aspects of the Japanese *amma*, or massage, were adapted and integrated with acupuncture concepts in a formal way to create the system of massage known as *shiatsu*. Massage was typically practiced by physicians and specialists. One problem that Japan faced with the expanded introduction of Chinese medicine was the difficulty of getting the raw materials. While many herbs in the Chinese pharmacopeia grew in Japan, many did not. Herbs such as cinnamon, rhubarb, and ephedra were difficult or impossible to cultivate in Japan and needed to be imported.

The result of this lack of access was that in many areas, Japanese folk medicine practices were, out of necessity, combined with Chinese herbal medicine. The scarcity of ingredients for the preparation of Chinese herbal formulas may have led to the lower doses typically seen in Japanese herbal prescriptions.

THE FIRST JAPANESE TEXT

In 982, Yasunari (Yasuyori) Tamba, a Japanese physician, composed a 30-volume compilation of medical knowledge at the direction of the emperor. His book *Ishinho* is considered the first Japanese medical text. It contains detailed discussions of the practice of *kanpo*, or Japanese herbal medicine. The text recommends acupuncture and moxibustion for many conditions. Based on Chinese medical theory, it quotes extensively from Chinese texts. It describes hygienic practices, acupuncture, moxibustion, magic, and many other topics, even the proper regulation of sexual activity.

BLIND ACUPUNCTURE AND GUIDE TUBES

In the seventeenth century, a blind man named Waichi Sugiyama began to train the blind in acupuncture using very fine needles and guide tubes. Sugiyama received a high official rank as an acupuncturist possibly as a result of successfully treating the Shogun (the military ruler of Japan). Since it had become customary in the earlier part of the Edo period for the blind to do massage, both massage and acupuncture now became associated with blind practitioners. This contributed in the long run to a lowering in the social position of acupuncture practitioners and to the further specialization in medical practice.

The guide tube that Sugiyama developed was a hollow metal cylinder that held the acupuncture needle upright against the skin. The tube allowed for finer needles to be inserted into the body and for needles to be inserted with less discomfort for the patients.

The prevalent use of fine needles and the guide tube continue to be distinctive features of Japanese acupuncture even today.

In modern Japan, both the blind and sighted continue to practice acupuncture, although as a result of Sugiyama's contribution, there are many schools of acupuncture for the blind.

The use of moxibustion was indicated for many conditions including the treatment of abscesses. Herbs, such as coptidis (*huang lian*), that we know today have marked antibiotic properties were recommended to treat infections.

GREATER INDEPENDENCE

The Kamakura period (1190–1333) saw the conclusion of a period of civil war with the establishment of a strong military rule. While the rulers in earlier periods had looked to China for guidance in the organization of the political world, this period revealed a distinctively Japanese approach to these matters.

Similarly, the Japanese physician began to show a greater independence in medical thought: Books and ideas continued to be imported from China, but these were now responded to more critically. According to the perspective of a contemporary acupuncturist, the practice of acupuncture and moxibustion began to decline in Japan. At the same time, moxibustion became part of the practices offered at Buddhist temples, and the knowledge of physicians (often *samurai*, or members of the privileged warriors class) became restricted to the feudal lords they served.

WESTERN EUROPE ENCOUNTERS JAPAN

In 1542, three Portuguese sailing on a Chinese junk were beached on Japan's shore by a typhoon. Within a few short years, seafaring Portuguese traders and Jesuit priests began to visit Japan with their minds set on trade and spiritual conquest. The Portuguese—and later the Spanish, Dutch, and Germans—established an extensive exchange of goods and ideas. Dutch and German physicians contributed ideas about medicine to the Japanese, and the Japanese exposed them to new ideas as well. "Dutch medicine," as western European practices came to be called in Japan, became increasingly important, culminating in an imperial decision to require that all doctors study Western medicine.

The political stability of the Edo period (1615–1867) supported a series of creative initiatives on the part of Japanese physicians. For example, guide tubes were developed to aid in the proper insertion of acupuncture needles. The Edo period also saw the continued introduction of Western medical ideas into Japan, especially anatomy. Medical knowledge continued to develop both through the independent efforts of Japanese physicians and through the arrival of new materials from China.

The philosophy and practice of medicine continued apace in various schools throughout this long period. The Koho School called for a return to older principles of therapy and diagnosis. Yoshimasu Todo (1720–1773)—a noted exponent of the Koho school—proposed that all disease resulted in poison being lodged in the body. He developed a system of abdominal diagnosis to assist in this task stating "The abdomen is the source of life and, therefore, the myriad diseases have their root here. The abdomen must always be examined in order to diagnose disease."

Another physician named Goto Gonzan (1659–1733) proposed the theory of *ikki-ryutai-setsu*, which suggested that the sole cause of disease was stagnation of *ki*. One pupil reports that he said "All diseases occur from the stagnation [of ki], and not from anything else. Wind and cold cause the stagnation [of ki], food and drinks cause the same, and seven kinds of emotions do the same, too. If the stagnation [of ki] takes place in one meridian or somewhere in the skin, it finally always infiltrates into the viscera."

What can be seen here is a characteristically Japanese desire to eliminate theoretical elaborations in favor of simple and practical therapeutic ideas.

One distinctive contribution to Japanese perspectives on diagnosis and therapy was made by a seventeenth century acupuncturist named Mubunsai. In 1685, he published a book called the *Compilation of the Secrets of Acupuncture,* which addressed the systematic diagnosis and treatment of disease through the abdomen. In his system, the abdomen was divided into specific regions, each associated with an organ. According to Mubunsai, the presence of evil ki can be felt in the abdomen, and where this is felt, the abdomen should be needled. Mubunsai developed a distinctive technique of *dashin,* in which a small wooden mallet was used to stimulate gold and silver needles that are held at the surface of the skin or slightly inserted.

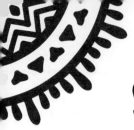

CENTRAL AND SOUTH AMERICA

THE AZTEC

Of all the great pre-Columbian civilizations, we know the most about the Aztec. We know about their statecraft, their gods and ceremonies, their art and architecture, their ideas about health and illness, their medicine men and medicinal plants, and all the other things that go into making a civilization, because we have several sources—some more reliable than others.

First, there were the chroniclers, the handful of Spanish friars with an inquiring bent of mind, who recorded what they saw and heard with accuracy and a degree of detachment even when what they were observing clashed with their deepest religious convictions. The greatest chronicler of them all was the Franciscan Fray Bernardino de Sahagún, author of the encyclopedic 12-volume *Historia General de las Cosas de Nueva España* (*General History of the Things of New Spain*), better known as the *Florentine Codex*.

Most of the early colonial writers were Mexican-born Spaniards, who approached Aztec medicine from the point of view of their own culture and religion. Exceptions are Sahagún and Martín de la Cruz, the author of the *Codex Badianus*, an illustrated treatise that lists over 250 Aztec medicinal plants and the ills for which they were employed. An additional 225 medicinal species are described in the *Florentine Codex*. However much these two works are relatively faithful to what the Aztec themselves said, they nevertheless show signs of careful editing, perhaps to avoid problems with the authorities.

Other sources, such as the monumental *Historia Natural* of Francisco Hernández, the learned physician to the king of Spain, owe much to European classifications, particularly the concept of humors and hot/cold dichotomies. Still, they provide additional information on the therapeutic uses of plants, animals, and minerals.

Of course there are holes in the record. On some aspects it is maddeningly vague. The early chroniclers inevitably saw the Aztec and their ways through the distorting lens of their own Spanish culture. There was much the chroniclers did not understand. There was much for which they had no model. And, being men as well as members of the clergy, they shut themselves off from women's culture and were, in turn, shut out by it. There was one inevitable conclusion from the writings of the chroniclers about Aztec medicine: In the year 1519, a patient had a much greater chance of dying under the ministrations of a Spanish physician than an Aztec doctor!

Finally, we also know more about the Aztec than other American civilizations because, at least in the countryside, so much of their culture, especially nutrition and medicine, endured through the colonial era into modern times; we can test the early writings against real life among the hundreds of thousands of villagers who still speak Nahuatl, the language of the Aztec, and dialects related to it.

BALANCED NUTRITION

Everywhere in the world, health and illness are directly linked to nutrition. It was no different for the Aztec, except that, as in China, the key was balance that was important. Foods considered to be "hot" or "warm" were especially beneficial because they added to the heat of your life force.

Local land supported two cultivated harvests a year. Each was an ecologic mini-universe that sustained a wide variety of foods other than the planted crops, such as migratory waterfowl, native birds, edible insects and their eggs, fish, shrimp, snakes, snails, and larval salamanders.

The salty waters of Lake Texcoco were also part of the Aztec food system, rich in nutritious, popular, and high-status foods, not the least of which were clusters of eggs laid by a corixid water beetle on pine branches the Aztec stuck in the muddy bottom of the shallow lake. Modern Indians still harvest them as "Mexican caviar" but use them to feed their songbirds rather than to enrich the dinner table as their Aztec ancestors did. More crucial still to Aztec nutrition and health was one of the world's true miracle foods: the edible one-celled, blue-green alga the Aztec called *tecuitlatl* (literally "excreta of stone"). Scientists identified it as *Spirulina geitlerii*. It attracted millions of migratory ducks, and the Aztec harvested great quantities of the floating mass in canoes, dried it in the sun, and traded it all over central Mexico in the form of flat, brick-shaped loaves the Spaniards said tasted like cheese. It remained for modern nutritionists to discover that an alga some modern writers thought had been no more than a "starvation food" actually contained all the essential amino acids and consisted of 70 percent protein of high biological quality, 18 percent carbohydrates, 8 percent fat, and many important vitamins and minerals, making this lowly one-celled lake product the nutritional equivalent of an egg. *Tecuitlatl* never found favor with the Spaniards, however, and it disappeared from the food trade when the Spaniards drained the lake to protect their capital against periodic flooding. One consequence of this loss of a great food source was the emergence of goiter as a chronic condition in parts of central Mexico, a condition the iodine in *tecuitlatl* had prevented.

As among other pre-Columbian peoples, Aztec medicine was a blend of the mystical and the practical. Religion, the calendar, divination, magic, and a relationship of mutual dependence between human beings and the gods all played a part in illness, as they did in curing. The practical consisted of close observation of the natural world and the response of symptoms to treatment by a vast array of medicinal plants, along with physical manipulations of the body and its organs.

Natural and Supernatural. Like other Native Americans, the Aztec made little distinction between "supernatural" and "natural" causes of disease, although the reality of natural causes—advanced age, for example—was recognized. "Supernatural," in the sense of something outside of, separate from, or, to use the literal meaning, "above" nature, is not part of Native American philosophy. There are realms of the stratified universe that are specific to certain kinds of spirits, such as sky gods and lords of the underworld, but otherwise the spirits are not conceived as apart from the natural world. Rather, they are integral to it. The spirits reside in, and manifest themselves as, natural phenomena that could be observed, touched, smelled, and so on.

If an Aztec physician divined a metaphysical cause for a given malady, it did not mean that it came from somewhere out there, beyond the physical world, beyond human understanding, and beyond the reach of empirical treatment. What it meant was that account must always be taken of the spiritual dimension in both illness and cure.

Tonalli. The Aztec world was full of spirits, according to the anthropologist and keen student of Aztec culture Bernard Ortiz de Montellano. Dangerous places and landmarks had "spirit owners," called *chaneques*, as did plants and animals. In addition to the gods, there were lesser spirits of clouds, trees, bushes, springs, crossroads, caves, rivers, lakes, mountains, even anthills. Since the Aztec universe was one of complementary oppositions, "owners" of water and earth were necessarily opposed to those of heat and sky, not as adversaries but as balanced counterparts. Human beings contained *tonalli*, the immaterial animating warmth that manifested itself especially in body heat and the blood coursing through the body. It was human *tonalli* that the spirits craved to strengthen themselves. The concept of *tonalli* (a word related to the Nahuatl *tona*, meaning "to make warm" or "sun") is extremely complex and would take an entire book to analyze and explain. The Aztec believed it entered the body only at the last moment before birth and left at death as the corpse turned cold. Another Aztec specialist, art historian Jill L. McKeever Furst, defines *tonalli* as the most important of the three souls possessed by each human being (the others being the *yolia* and the *ihiyotl*). Too much or too little of any of these causes illness, but *tonalli* is the most important.

Tonalli extends outward from the individual into the universe and inward from the universe into the body, where one feels it in one's flesh as warmth and pumping blood. It manifests itself in the heat of sunshine and the glow of fire, which is why the patient should be placed close to a fire or exposed to the warming rays of the sun. Postmenopausal women are especially rich in *tonalli*, manifesting itself, among other ways, in the phenomenon of hot flashes. The problem for humans was that the spirits of nature were forever trying to absorb *tonalli*, for example, by drawing it out from people incautious enough to approach them in an inappropriate manner. Loss of *tonalli* meant a potentially fatal weakening. Its cure required correct diagnosis, starting with the identification of the offended spirit and the determination of the cause of his or her displeasure.

Ehecames. Loss of one's animating life force—the weakening, misplacement, or abduction of the *tonalli*—was taken to be one major cause of sickness. Another was "sickness intrusion," meaning the magical invasion of the body by a disease-carrying object. This, in turn, was closely related to the idea of "bad winds," the *ehecames* that survive today as the *mal aires* of Mexican folk belief.

Usually the injection into the body of a foreign disease-carrying object was diagnosed as the work of a disgruntled ancestor or deity, displeased at having been ignored or insufficiently honored with gifts, or as the evil deed of a shaman in the employ of a human enemy. With everything animate, even a tool might avenge itself in this way on its owner if not treated with respect and given food in a ceremony devoted to this duty. The *ehecames* could enter the body through orifices, manifesting themselves as worms, hair, or some other foreign object, and make the person sick. A major source of these ill winds were the restless souls of the recently departed. There were many other sources of dangerous *ehecames*: the earth itself, the underworld, water, hills, and caves.

MEDICAL SPECIALISTS

Treating illness often required a two-pronged approach. Recovery of the soul (*tonalli*) and extraction of the pathogen (*ehecames*) by sucking directly into the mouth of the shaman or through a tube were in the realm of religion and magic. The treatment of the actual symptoms was not, although those who did the curing operated in both the metaphysical and the physical realms.

There was a whole range of specialists. Built into each practitioner was his opposite, the "good" shaman to cure, the "bad" shaman to make ill. Whether that was how his consultants explained it or the only way he could make sense of what they told him is difficult to say. Perhaps the antagonistic, or complementary, qualities were really present in the same individual. There was, first, the *naualli*. The Spaniards translated it as "sorcerer." We would call him a shaman.

A second class of healer, similarly separated into good and bad, read the day's divinatory signs in the 260-day calendar for their negative or positive aspects and revealed the truth to the clients. Finally there is the physician, *ticitl* in Na-huatl, whom the *Florentine Codex* describes as a curer of people and a restorer and provider of health:

The good physician [is] a diagnostician, experienced—a knower of herbs, of stones, of trees, of roots. He has [results of] examinations, experience, prudence. [He is] moderate in his acts. He provides health, restores people, provides them splints, sets bones for them, purges them, gives emetics, gives them potions; he lances, he makes incisions in them, stitches them, revives them, envelops them in ashes.

And then there is his opposite:

The bad physician [is] a fraud, a halfhearted worker, a giver of overdoses, an in-creaser [of sickness]; one who endangers others, who worsens sickness, who causes one to worsen. [He pretends to be] a counselor, advised, chaste. He bewitches; he is a sorcerer, a soothsayer, a caster of lots, a diagnostician by means of knots. He kills with his medicines; he increases [sickness]; he seduces women, he bewitches them.

DIAGNOSIS BY HALLUCINATION

There was overlap among the various practitioners of the shamanic and medi-cal arts, just as there was between the spiritual, the pragmatic, and experiential in Aztec medical science. For divination and diagnosis, probably every kind of curer resorted to ritual hallucinogens, including:

- the peyote cactus
- *ololiuhqui*—the seeds of the morning glory *Turbina corymbosa*, which contain ergot alkaloids
- species of the *Datura* and *Solandra genii* (from the nightshade family)
- the sacred mushrooms, which contain the hallucinogen psilocybin

The respect accorded to the sacred psilocybin mushroom is self-evident from what the Aztec called them: *teonanácatl*, meaning "flesh of the gods."

MEDICINES

We are blessed with a great number of sources on how the Aztec saw and treated disease. There are lists of virtually every ailment known to the Indians, each with its corresponding medicinal plants. Most of the plants have been identified; the number tested by modern methods is small but growing steadi-ly. The therapeutic effect the Aztec claimed for them has not been confirmed for some, but for others, for which pharmacologic information is available, the results are favorable, attesting to the high state of Aztec empirical medicine.

The plants traditionally used in Mexico for the treatment of dental disease provide a case in point. Aztec healers and their successors employed 107 species for 17 different oral conditions:

- 27 plants for the treatment of thrush, among them the psychotropic peyote cactus, *Lophophora williamsii* (which is known to contain antibiotics effective against several kinds of infections), and several popular ornamentals, such as cosmos, geranium, heliotrope, hibiscus, and bromelia
- 8 plants for local anesthesia, including extracts of croton and species of the pepper family
- 42 plants for toothache, among them three species of tobacco
- 7 plants for dental decay
- 5 for gum disease
- 4 for halitosis (bad breath)
- 10 for gingivitis
- 15 for inflammation of the mouth

Only a fraction of these have been tested, but ten have yielded highly favorable results. It is interesting that in the treatment of thrush, the native doctors also discovered the healing properties of two species of plantain, *Plantago mexicana* and *Plantago lanceolatum*. The latter, and its broad-leaved sister species, *Plantago major*, were also used by Native North Americans, as well as by Europeans since at least the Middle Ages, to speed the healing of cuts, running sores, and other wounds.

THE MAYA

To us, the Maya are perhaps the most mysterious of the great pre-Columbian civilizations. Whereas the Spanish encountered an Aztec civilization at the height of its imperial power, the Maya flourished long before the Europeans even knew a Western Hemisphere existed. It is hard enough to determine the monumental events of the later part of the Maya civilization, much less piece together the details of everyday living during the height of the Classic period. There are some excellent sources from the years around the time of the arrival of the Spanish—remarkably detailed and accurate documentation on the afflictions that plagued people and on the plants the shamans employed against them—but for the millennia of Maya settlement in Yucatán prior to the 1500s, there is nothing; and there are few, if any, reliable accounts for the southern part of the Maya territory.

RECONSTRUCTING MAYA MEDICINE

That all the written information comes from Yucatán just prior to, and just after, the European invasion does not tie our hands completely. It is probably safe to assume that Yucatecan Maya medicine in the early colonial period applies as well to earlier times and other places. There was clearly considerable stability to the medical prescriptions of the Maya physicians, for even those written after two centuries of European influence show little alteration from those that date to the 1500s. So perhaps we can push some of these medical practices at least back to the glory days of Classic Maya civilization.

Thanks to recent advances in the reading of many of the hieroglyphic texts carved on Maya monuments and painted on pottery, we have learned a good deal about dynastic succession, warfare, conquest, alliances between rival city-states, and the dates when these events occurred.

In contrast to all this knowledge we could not have dreamed of possessing a few decades ago, everyday Maya life is still a great big blank. We know nothing from the written and painted sources about the one thing that must have most concerned the average citizens of the cities and mini-empires of the Classic period, just as it concerns them and us today: their health. Skeletal remains tell us something of nutritional stress and disease but, except for healed fractures, provide no firsthand evidence of treatment or its effectiveness.

THE LORD'S CACAO CUP

In the tombs of some nobles and rulers were found elegant cylindrical vases. Some of these works of art have turned out to be nothing less than chocolate drinking cups, their hieroglyphic texts proclaiming, "This is the chocolate drinking cup of Lord . . ." followed by the name of the owner.

The foamy drink the Maya brewed from the crushed and partially fermented fatty seeds of the cacao tree (*Theobroma cacao*) was an important ceremonial food. And, as with the Aztec and the South Americans, the same plants that figured in ritual or triggered the shamanic state of altered consciousness also had a therapeutic dimension. Cacao was no exception.

The active principle in cacao seeds is theobromine, a bitter alkaloid related to caffeine. Like caffeine, theobromine is an addictive, or at least habit-forming, stimulant. Modern chemistry has confirmed that theobromine also has a protective effect by inhibiting bacteria like *Streptococcus*, *Shigella*, *Staphylococcus*, and other assorted pathogens that, among other ill effects on human health, contribute to tooth decay. The precise pharmacology would not have been known by the Maya shaman, but the effects told the story.

Cacao beans have a high content of fat, and this the Maya physician extracted and applied to wounds and infections to speed the process of healing, while an infusion that concentrated theobromine was employed as a diuretic to increase the flow of urine. Chocolate as medicine—it seems we have a lot to learn from the Maya.

Still, "nothing" may be too broad a term. On rare occasions, we can infer something from what the ancient artists painted on funerary pottery. Almost everyone of high status, especially rulers and their close relatives, was buried with an array of food bowls and ceremonial ceramics. Some are plain, many richly decorated. Most of this art does not bother with daily concerns. Painted vessels depict mythologic events or someone's out-of-body experiences, a mystical encounter, perhaps, between the companion spirit of the deceased and the denizens of other worlds, or a ritual dance in company with the spirits of ancestors and sacred animals. Still, the ancient artists' subject matter is not all beyond our understanding. Sometimes it is almost embarrassingly frank.

SPIRITS AND OFFERINGS

Maya conception and treatment of illness drew equally on religion, magic, and science. The Maya believed that death, disease, and other physical and emotional afflictions were almost always punishment for wrongdoings. Before a cure could be attempted, the healer had to discover the identity of whatever spirit the patient might have offended or neglected, and what actions, practical and metaphysical, were required to reverse the victim's ill fortune. However, once that was out of the way, depending on the nature of the affliction, the practical could come into play. Chief among offenses that could make people sick, requiring the services of the healer, was failure to honor and give sustenance to the gods and ancestors with offerings of ceremonial foods. Suitable gifts included:

- heart-shaped cakes molded of maize or pumpkin seeds
- the smoke of burning tobacco and balls of rubber
- perfuming the ground with incense and maize before the sacred idols carved of wood or stone
- human sacrifice (on special occasions)

NATURAL MEDICINES

Whatever "magical thinking" went into Maya medical beliefs (and there was quite a bit), there was much that was clearly practical and effective. The colonial medical literature enumerates a wide range of species we now know exhibit broad-spectrum antimicrobial activity, for example. So, if some Maya remedies suggest "superstition," the many detailed descriptions of plants used in Maya medicine confirm that there was as much that was empirical and systematic. The point is not whether there was a religious or magical component to Maya medical practice; it is that the Maya had a broader concept of naturopathy than we do. The healing power of plants came from and belonged to the realm of the spirits. As in South America today, certain species were identified as plant deities and teachers of herbal expertise. For the medicine to work, the shaman had to give it its proper psychological and spiritual dimension.

There was no shortage of medicinal plants or of expertise in their effects. In 1931, the scholar Ralph L. Roys was able to discern 447 separate medical conditions, together with their corresponding herbal prescriptions and other therapeutic techniques. For asthma, the medical tracts prescribed the crushed leaves and bark of *Coc-che* (*Conocarpus erecta*, or button tree; also called *boton-cillo* in rural Mexico). Among the several cures for blood in the urine was an astringent tonic made from, among other healing plants:

- the bark of *chim-tok* (*Krugiodendron ferreum*, or black ironwood; also called *Quiebra hacha* in Spanish), a hardwood tree with dull green leaves
- the *plumilla* (*Trixis radialis*, called *hierba del aire* in Spanish)
- *sanguinaria de flores negro*, roughly meaning "the one with the black flow-ers that is thirsty for blood" (*Sanvitalia procumbens*, or creeping zinnia)
- the leaves, stalks, and root of *Melochia tomentosa* and *Cenchrus echinatus*

Some of these were also used for a variety of other ills, alone or in combi-nation. So, for example, *Trixis radialis*, another species of the same genus as *Trixis inula*, has 12 different medical uses, internal and external, including those for open sores, edema, swollen feet, and pneumonia.

An important beverage in Maya ritual was *balché*, an alcoholic drink made of fermented honey and an extract of the bark of the purplish-flowered *balché* tree (*Lonchocarpus longistylus*). It may have figured in enema rites as well. The Maya medical texts prescribe the crushed leaves of the tree as a poultice for smallpox (a disease unknown in the Americas before the European invasion) and an infusion to cure loss of speech. Many Maya still use the *balché* drink today ceremonially, recreationally, and medicinally.

The intoxicating morning glory seeds the Maya call *xtabentun* were also used as medicine, possibly in enemas. Morning glories are plentiful in their envi-ronment, especially along stream and river beds, and we know they used the seeds. There is no information on *xtabentun* as a hallucinogen, but one of the earliest Maya medicinal texts credits it with beneficial effects in, among other ailments, kidney stones and disorders of the urinary tract.

THE INCA

The Inca empire was a vast multiethnic state, stretching for thousands of miles along the west coast of South America. A technologically and administratively advanced civilization, they built an impressive highway system—over 15,000 miles of roads—along the coastal desert and high in the Andes Mountains. The Inca, like the Aztec and the Maya, also eventually fell to the invading Spanish, but not before they had developed a culture—and a medical tradition—as rich as any other in the Americas.

THE KALLAWAYAS, HEALERS OF THE ANDES

There are still some 13,000 people in and around La Paz, Bolivia, that are called *Kallawayas*. They are not of the same ethnic stock as the Inca, and they were probably originally speakers of a dialect of Aymara (the language of most Bolivian Indians) not Quechua (the language of the Inca and of many Peruvian Indians today). *Kallawaya* literally means "Land of the Medicine," and these natives have given us a good look at what medicine was like during the days of the empire.

Five hundred years ago, the Kallawayas played a key role in Inca medicine, in trade between the highlands and the tropical lowlands, and in the expansion and consolidation of the empire. They were considered by the Inca rulers to be the direct descendants of the Sun. It was their role as healers and herbalists to be the bearers of all Inca rulers and other nobles as they traveled across their far-flung empire and into unknown territory, just as a doctor accompanies the president of the United States on all his travels.

The Kallawayas descended regularly from the highlands of the Andes to the tropical jungle, where they gathered their medicinal herbs to take back and treat the sick. (They continue to do so to this day.) They were still at the beginning of this century taking their healing herbs and their knowledge all through the Andean nations: Bolivia, Chile, Ecuador, Peru, and Argentina—all the places that once came under Inca influence.

A few years ago there was a lucky archaeologic discovery in Kallawaya territory: an undisturbed medicine man's grave dating from AD 400, a time when the Andean culture was rapidly expanding. The male occupant of the grave was accompanied by a typical shaman's kit: carved wooden snuff tablets and tubes; a gourd container with remains of an hallucinogenic snuff powder; leaves from a species of holly (*Ilex guayusa*); a trephined skull; and enema syringes, one consisting of a hollow reed with a bulb of animal intestine tied to it with cotton string.

Holly. Tea brewed from *Ilex guayusa* and its sister species, *Ilex paraguariensis*, is still drunk in great quantities by many South American people. It is used as a pick-me-up in the morning, to relieve fatigue after heavy labor or long journeys, and to settle the stomach or calm the nerves. Kallawayas also use preparations made from this and related plants for sunburn, to reduce inflammation, and to cleanse and dry infected wounds. The leaves accompanying our ancient Kallawaya shaman were carefully prepared in groups of three and five for his final journey. No one knows the uses to which the ancient shaman put his leaves, but there is little question that he and his contemporaries recognized their healthful properties.

Trephination. Trephination is a surgical procedure of which there is ancient evidence found in most parts of the world. It involves the drilling of a small hole or holes in the skull to relieve pressure or allow illness out. The trephined skull found in the shaman's grave is the earliest evidence we have for skull surgery in the Andes. The traditional procedure had become almost extinct in the Andes early in this century, but from this ancient grave, it seems it was already highly developed by AD 400. The skull found with the medicine man had three openings drilled with flint or obsidian, for what reason we do not know. However, we do know that the patient survived; the bone around the openings shows signs of healing.

The art of trephining became highly developed in Inca times, probably because of the need to repair damage from war clubs to the heads of warriors during their conquest of more than 5,000 miles of mountainous territory in the 100 years before the Spanish conquest. (Some of the ancient Mexicans, too, made successful use of trephining, as shown by, among other evidence, skulls found at Monte Alban, Oaxaca, on which the bone had grown back around the surgical openings.)

Enemas. Medicinal enemas also have a long history in the Andes. Early in this century, some Andean shamans were reported to be still using enemas with infusions of psychoactive plants to enhance their spirit powers. The type of enema apparatus found in the shaman's grave also occurs among the Amazonian Indians and has a history in Peru, at least as far back as the first century AD.

A WEALTH OF BOTANICAL KNOWLEDGE

The Spanish conquistadors were impressed by the wealth of medicinal plants known to Peruvian healers and attempted to obtain as much information on them as possible, without regard to the natives' magical explanations of their effectiveness. Even though purification and public confession of transgressions, such as neglect of ancestor worship, was widely considered essential to a cure, the early chroniclers mention only native decoctions made from the plant kingdom for numerous common afflictions, from rheumatism and flux to depression, epilepsy, dropsy, and scabies. Indeed, the discoveries of the medicinal properties of plants by Andean and lowland South American Indians have resulted in some of the most dramatic improvements in modern therapeutics.

Where would surgery be without the coca plant, *Erythroxylon coca*, a cultivated native of the Amazon basin and the Andes, which some native peoples held, and still hold, to be holy? The plant—the source of cocaine—is not known in a completely wild state; it has been cultivated and used against numerous conditions, including altitude sickness, hunger, fatigue, sore throat, and stomach and intestinal ills and for increasing the nutritional value of a high-starch diet. These uses date back at least 2,000 years and probably before that.

Modern medicine uses countless medicines—or, more precisely, synthetic versions of them—that were commonplace in the Andes. Ipecac, curare, sassafras, cascara, and balsam now have their synthetic equivalents but are still important in modern medicine. Essential oils, alkaloids, flavonoids, saponins, and other chemicals have been isolated from *Chenopodium linneus* and its sister species, from which South Americans decoct effective purgatives and vermifuges. One species, *Chenopodium quinoa*, is the source of a nutritious Andean seed crop available in many health food stores. Nor must we forget tobacco—one of the most prominent and most sacred plants in South American shamanism that also has a major role in native therapeutics, especially as a fumigant.

Finally there is quinine, the most effective of all remedies for malaria—indeed, the most important medicinal plant Peru gave to the world. Therein lies an interesting story. Quinine is an alkaloid extract from the bark of the *cinchona* tree or shrub mentioned in the seventeenth century Spanish colonial literature as *arbol de calentura*, or "fever tree." The first Europeans to describe *cinchona* were struck by the fact that the Indian people not only professed ignorance of its antimalarial qualities but refused to take it. Nor did the Kallawayas know anything about it. The reason, of course, was not some sort of "blind spot" in native plant therapeutics, but the fact that malaria was one of those dreadful foreign scourges the Europeans introduced into the Americas.

Public Health. Perhaps the most noteworthy aspect of Inca medicine was their public health policy. Herbalists and other healers received public remuneration, and the poor and disabled were fed from communal lands. There was a law that every surgeon and other nonherbal medical specialist should be fully trained in medicinal plant lore. A kind of genetic engineering was practiced, in that congenitally malformed individuals were required to marry only among themselves. Houses were well constructed against heat, cold, and vermin, and cities were supplied with ample and healthful water. People who failed to observe hygiene regulations were publicly excoriated and subject to penalties. Diet and work were highly regulated, and although whole populations were transplanted by the totalitarian Inca regime, attention was paid to the association between health, climate, and altitude.

Finally, the fundamentally social and religious attitude toward health was confirmed by the annual public celebration of a great prophylactic ritual, known as *citua*. It was held in September at the onset of the rainy season, which was regarded as the season of disease. On this occasion, the statues of the deities were paraded around the Inca capital, after which the emperor dispatched four parties of warriors to the four directions to drive out the disease spirits. The entire population, meanwhile, shook the demons of illness out of their clothes and took part in ritual bathing and fumigation with tobacco smoke, coating their faces and houses with a sacred paste made from ground maize.

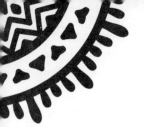

NORTH AMERICA

Describing the healing traditions of Native North Americans is not as simple as describing those of, say, the ancient Egyptians. The people that inhabited the continent before the arrival of the Europeans came during three different migrations from at least three different areas of Asia, each with different traditions. Over a period of at least 12,000 years, they spread down and across the continent, adapting and developing hundreds of different cultures, as rich and varied as the lands the people came to inhabit—from the soggy, wooded Northwest Coast to the forests of upstate New York to the desert of the Great Basin.

Many tribes did use similar methods; shamanism, herbal remedies, healing ceremonies, and other forms of spiritual healing seem to be found in most North American tribes. However, different underlying beliefs led to an amazing array of approaches.

SPIRIT DANCING AMONG THE SALISH

The spirit dance of the Salish of northern Washington and southern British Columbia is called the *Tamanawas*. The word is a corruption of *tomanoas*, meaning "guardian spirit" in Cowitchan, one of the indigenous languages of the Northwest Coast. The word became shorthand for the spirit dance. As its name implies, one of its purposes was acquisition of a guardian spirit who would stand at your side and help you through life's crises and illness. The idea of a guardian spirit can be found in virtually every Native American culture, but in British Columbia and northern Washington it took a much more dramatic and public form.

The spirit dance involves a severe psychological and physical trauma in which the patient is "killed" before he or she can be reborn, recharged with spirit power, and healed. Centuries old and nearly extinguished during years of official repression, the Salish rite has proved its modern worth in treating drug and alcohol addiction, depression, and other ailments of the spirit, which are aggravated, if not actually caused, by the relative deprivation, discrimination, unemployment, colonialism, hopelessness, anger, and other negatives of modern Native American life.

One aim of the dance was recovery of personal spirit power, the loss of which made one vulnerable to invasion by disease agents. This loss of spirit power might even lead to death. A man or woman could lose personal spirit power through inappropriate behavior toward family or community, an encounter with and possession by a hostile spirit, or even the inadvertent acquisition of the wrong kind of spirit song—a ritual song associated with certain spiritually derived powers.

Spirit dancing is drastic medicine. Preparation of participants can take weeks of purification and psychic and physical training. It means fasting to the point of hallucination, seclusion in total darkness, alternate periods of sensory deprivation and overload, instruction in tribal lore and community values, physical and psychological pressure, and, most dramatically, the initiate's symbolic death by "clubbing," also called "doctoring up" or "grabbing."

Usually this leads to temporary loss of consciousness. Taken together, these ordeals have the purpose of personality depatterning and reorientation, intended to make the initiate forget and abandon his or her former self and shortcomings. The initiate falls into the kind of ecstatic trance that is one of the universal characteristics of the shamanic journey. In this altered state of consciousness, the spirit dancer travels to the underworld, the land of the ancestral dead. In the process he or she acquires a spirit song, new self-knowledge, and the restoration or enhancement of personal spirit power that may have become lost or weakened.

Already shaken to the core in anticipation, the candidate spirit dancer is kept in the longhouse, secluded in a dark cubicle, or "smokehouse tent," for a period of usually ten days, which may be reduced to four days or prolonged for several weeks or even the whole season. The length of this seclusion seems to depend mainly on the novice's motivation and his conscious or unconscious cooperation in "finding his song and dance," which is the professed purpose of the initiation process.

The principal therapeutic functions of this process—personality depatterning and reorientation—are not unknown to the ritualists. In the words of a senior participant:

It is an Indian treatment, it is a kind of brainwashing, four to ten days of torture. Through this torture they soften up; their brains get soft. During this time you're the weakest and your brain is back to nil; anything you are taught during those ten days is going to stick with you; you're never going to forget it. There is always someone with you during that time, always telling you to change your life. This is when you are taught all rules of your culture . . . the harder the torture, the stronger you get.

Or, as one Salish man put it

They kill you as an evil person. They revive you to a new human being. That's why when they club you, you just go out and pass out, but you come back . . . There is not to be evil thinking after they are through with you, all you think is, I'm starting life all over again.

The spirit journey of the novice reenacts a familiar drama: A shaman travels to the land of the dead to recover the lost or stolen soul of his patient and return it to the land of the living and the healthy. In the Salish version of this virtually universal shamanic experience, the shaman makes his journey in a spirit canoe. He faces west on his way to the underworld, and east on his return to the land of the living. When he has located the soul and placed it in his canoe he poles as hard as he can upriver against a fast-flowing current "toward light and life."

In fact, this essential element of shamanic practice—traveling to other worlds to recover abducted or otherwise lost souls—is implicit in the Salish word for shaman, which in English roughly translates to "the one who travels."

The shaman's canoe journey to recover the soul from the realm of the dead used to be reenacted in Salish ceremonialism. Playing himself, the shaman would carry a long magical pole which he manipulated like a canoe pole or paddle. This aspect of Salish shamanism survives mainly in the spirit journey of the novices and of mature spirit dancers who repeat the therapeutic experience every year during the winter ceremonies.

Between their symbolic death and rebirth, the novices are conceived of as "babies" unable to fend for themselves. They are given special protective clothing or "uniforms," a staff, and "babysitters" who help keep them safe along the way. Like newborn babies, but also like the shamans on their trance journeys to the Land of the Dead, the novices are very vulnerable.

Traveling in an altered state of consciousness that simulates death, they must overcome numerous obstacles and resist all manner of temptations, such as foodstuffs offered to them by the spirits—an especially difficult ordeal after their long fasts. They also emulate the shaman on his spirit canoe journey by wielding their staffs to "pole themselves upstream" toward the land of the living. But they can return fully to earthly existence only when they have achieved their goal: the acquisition of their healing songs, guardian spirits, and personal spirit power.

SPIRIT ILLNESS

A condition known as "spirit illness" that does not yield to scientific medicine also plays an important role across the entire area of northwestern North America where spirit dancing was practiced. This seasonal condition is akin to another shamanic phenomenon—initiatory illness, or "sickness vocation." Initiatory illness is supernatural recruitment of a candidate to the shamanic profession by gods, spirits, or ancestor shamans.

The advent of the winter season, with its spirit dances, is heralded by the visible sickening of all those who have acquired the will and the power to dance. They become distraught, anxious, depressed, despondent, anorexic, emaciated, and weak, and they suffer local and general pains. These conditions require the intervention of experienced shamans as mediating therapists, but they may also yield to the sympathetic ministrations of experienced spirit dancers and members of the community.

THE FALSE-FACE SOCIETY

Among the greatest works of Native North American artists are the masks that Alaskan Eskimos, the Salish of northern Washington and southern British Columbia, the Tlingit of Alaska, and the Haida, Tsimshians, Kwakiutl, Bella Coola, and other indigenous peoples of the Pacific Northwest made to represent animal spirits and ancestors in ceremonies. But 3,000 miles to the east, the Iroquois of upstate New York and the Canadian province of Ontario have an old masking tradition that for centuries has been a crucial element in traditional doctoring.

Medicine "Faces" representing spirit beings continue to be carved of basswood by men who dance to the sound of turtle-shell rattles in dramatic midwinter rites to drive away disease, purify houses, and cure their occupants. The women of these matrilineal societies, meanwhile, braid another kind of forest and vegetation spirit face of dried cornhusk.

The curing function of the masks comes into play not only in the midwinter ceremonial and other seasonal observances but at any time of the year when someone dreams of a mask and feels the need of a cure by a member of the Society of Faces.

Following a successful cure, the dreamer may himself join the Society; most of its members join after seeing a "face" in a dream and being healed by it. A new member may ask an experienced carver to make a mask for him or her representing the spirit that appeared in his or her dream. But owning a mask is not a requirement. Many members, in fact, borrow masks from friends to participate in a curing rite.

Some masks depict animals, but most represent mythologic beings that appeared to the Iroquois in ancient times while hunting or gathering food or, more recently, in a dream. With their sometimes grotesquely distorted features, long manes of horsehair, and shiny metal rings around the eyes, the "faces" are not intended to disguise the wearer but to give substance to ephemeral beings the hunters might have seen flitting from tree to tree or hiding beneath waterfalls and rocks.

WHIRLWIND

The power of some masks goes far beyond individual or communal curing. Suspended from trees in the forest, or even thrown into the face of an approaching storm, they are believed capable of turning away blizzards and tornadoes. There is an old tale told by the Cayuga, another of the Iroquois peoples, that accounts for the origin of the first mask of Whirlwind—a spirit so dangerous that even such powerful beings as Lightning and Thunder failed to strike him down. The story recalls a sickness that can be cured only by the patient's agreeing to become a shaman:

One day a hunter stalking game with a companion in the forest inadvertently glimpsed the face of the Whirlwind spirit. Blood began to spurt from his nose and when it would not stop, he fell over dead. The second man was luckier, escaping with his life even though he, too, saw the Whirlwind face peering at him from behind a tree. Back in the village he asked a shaman to divine what had happened to him and his friend. He was instructed to return to the forest with a tobacco offering for the Whirlwind spirit. In this way he would himself become a curer.

The man returned to the forest with his offerings, but try as he might, the man failed to get another glimpse of the Whirlwind face. At last he fell into a deep sleep, and in his dream he saw a man carving a Whirlwind mask intended for him. When he awakened he sought out the carver and obtained the mask. A few nights later his wife dreamed of a terrible approaching storm that would surely kill them unless her husband hung the mask from a tree and burned a tobacco offering to Whirlwind. The storm passed over them without harm, and in gratitude, the man, now a full-fledged curing shaman, carved the spirit's likeness in three sizes: one life-size to be worn in the curing ceremonies, a second smaller one to be carried for protection, and a third in miniature. This one he suspended from the largest mask as its companion.

In fact, miniature replicas of the larger masks serve some vital functions. They can be substituted for their life-size prototypes and they are thought to protect their owners against illness just as well as the full-size masks. They are also thought to be effective in curing their owners from troubling dreams caused by a hostile Mask Spirit.

Cures of this kind are part of the so-called dream-guessing ritual that was traditionally held during the midwinter ceremony. The dream-guessing ritual was first described by French Jesuit missionaries, who were astonished by the sophistication with which the Iroquois treated emotional ills, their understanding of unconscious causes, and the effectiveness of the treatment prescribed by the elders. As anthropologists have pointed out, the Iroquois's dream-guessing rite was a primitive but very effective form of psychotherapy that recognized, long before Freud, the latent and manifest content of dreams.

ANCIENT BUT STILL LIVING

How old is the Iroquois tradition of representing forest spirits with wooden masks and using them to drive away disease spirits and restore individuals and the group to health? No one can say. During the American Revolution, the Iroquois allied themselves with the British, from whose colonial officials they had received greater respect and better treatment than from the Yankee settlers. The result was scorched-earth destruction of the Iroquois's crops and villages and, with the American defeat of the British, dismemberment and alienation of much of their traditional land in New York. Out of the ashes of defeat came spiritual rebirth with the new religion of the Longhouse, a blending of older pre-European indigenous beliefs with the reformist message of the Seneca prophet Handsome Lake. Ever since, the society of the curing masks and its traditions and rituals have been firmly embedded in the Longhouse Religion.

But like the Iroquois Longhouse itself, mask healing in Iroquois culture is clearly much older. One authority was convinced that the masks and their ritual context belong to a very ancient woodlands tradition. Miniature "faces" similar to the life-size masks are modeled on clay tobacco pipes dating back to the 1500s. This suggests an antiquity reaching at least as far back as late pre-colonial times, some 500 years ago. As for the cornhusk masks that mainly depict vegetation spirits, corn, or maize, these originated many millennia ago in Mexico. It reached the Iroquois about 1,000 years ago, along with *Nicotiana rustica* tobacco, a South American hybrid first cultivated, along with its sister species *Nicotiana tabacum*, perhaps 7,000 years ago on the eastern slopes of the Andes. The Iroquois still tie small bundles of *Nicotiana rustica* to the masks and burn them as sacred offerings to the spirits the masks represent.

To the Iroquois, the masks are not objects of worship. They are alive, capable like any human being of seeing, hearing, and feeling, so much so that when not in use, they are supposed to be kept lying facedown and wrapped up lest they see and hear things that might offend them. They are not art for art's sake, carved to decorate the home or fill out a museum exhibit. Rather they make visible and concrete the ephemeral spirit beings that are very real and sacred to the Iroquois.

Their representations in wood and cornhusk are imbued with a beneficent life force not unlike that attributed to the several hundred medicinal plants that continue to play a role in traditional Iroquois healing.

Likewise, dancing with the mask in the midwinter rites is not a nostalgic reenactment of an ancient shamanistic curing ritual that has lost its meaning in the face of modern medicine. It is a living tradition in every sense. The masks are not the icons of a bygone faith, but a central and vital component of an ancient art of healing the spirit when it is most in need of community support and sustenance.

THE HEALING HERBS OF THE CHIPPEWA

It is often said that the indigenous peoples of North America were in touch with their natural environments to an extent unknown to the peoples of Europe. Certainly in the realm of medicine and, particularly, the use of botanical medicine, Native North American peoples had an extensive knowledge. North American Indians put to use thousands of unique plants and their different parts—roots, flowers, stems, seeds, leaves—in the internal and external treatment of hundreds of ailments, from snakebite and skin rash to hepatitis and broken limbs.

Although medicinal herbs play a part in the Salish spirit dance and the Iroquois had extensive herbal pharmacies, medicinal flora really came into its own among the Chippewa and other Algonquin-speaking adherents of the now-defunct Midewiwin, or Grand Medicine Society. It was in their initiations into the several grades of the shamanistic Mide organization that initiates acquired expertise in the therapeutic properties of plants. The other side of the coin was that the natural world also provided the means to make people sick and to kill. This dangerous knowledge was also among the secrets imparted to the initiates into the Midewiwin, contributing to the suspicion and hostility it fostered over time and its ultimate demise.

The number of medicinal plants used by the first Americans is so vast it defies counting. In 1977, a book called *American Medical Botany: A Reference Dictionary* listed 1,288 different species belonging to 531 genera in 118 different families employed in 48 different cultures. Two additional studies done in the 1970s—one on the medicinal plants of the Cherokee by Paul B. Hamel and Mary U. Chiltoskey and a doctoral dissertation on the medical botany of the Iroquois by James W. Herrick—added more than 4,000. Thousands more have since been added to the list.

Significantly, no matter how distant from one another in geography, language, and culture, the healers of some of these indigenous populations often hit on the same or closely related species for similar ailments. These similarities arose even in the absence of contact, leading to the conclusion that healers probably used close observation and experimentation—empirical methods—to develop their herbal pharmacies.

LEVELS OF MIDEWIWIN

The Midewiwin, or Grand Medicine Society, was a secret society open to both men and women among such Algonquin-speaking eastern woodlands peoples as the Chippewa (or Ojibway), Ottawa, Sauk, Fox, Winnebago, Potawatomie, and Kickapoo. It was divided into four grades in ascending rank order, and its members, dressed in festive clothing, met in a specially constructed lodge to dance, make offerings, and pray to different *manidos*, under the leadership of initiated Mide priests. The society was named for a magical white shell, *mide* in the indigenous language, which members newly initiated into the first grade were taught to control and use to "shoot" into other members, as it had been shot into themselves, to give them sacred power.

Acceptance into the different grades involved payment by the initiate who, in turn, was presented with the skins of mink, otter, fish, and other animals and a special medicine bag in which he or she kept the magical shell. Those newly initiated were also taught the properties of medicinal plants and how to cure with them. Over time this special knowledge came to be so feared as sorcery and witchcraft by nonmembers that the Grand Medicine Society fell into disrepute and was even outlawed; their initiations were stopped by one group after another.

Only memories survive of the Mide among the Indian people of the Great Lakes region. But in its glory days, its origin was credited to none other than the divine hero and sometime trickster known variously as Manabozho, Mänabush, Nanabozho, or Winnebajo. According to the story of the Mide, the sky gods gave the hero the Grand Medicine lodge and its secrets to comfort him after the underwater *manidos* killed his younger brother and inseparable companion Little Wolf. (In Great Lakes native mythology, the underwater monsters were the sworn enemies of the Thunderbirds, the *manidos* of the sky.)

The hero brought the medicine lodge down to earth from the sky and taught human beings the Mide secrets so that they might cure disease, defeat their enemies, and enjoy a long and healthy life and abundant foodstuffs. These included wild rice, an important staple that was eaten seasoned with maple sugar or combined with duck or venison broth.

Among the hundreds of plants used as medicine by the Chippewa, at least 69 have been identified and recognized by whites for their medicinal value, including several that made it into various editions of the United States Pharmacopoeia (USP). Others have been accepted by at least some physicians or long been used as family remedies by Europeans who had settled near or in the native communities. Some examples include:

Seneca snakeroot (*Polygala senega L.*)—The roots were used as a decoction for coughs and colds and the leaves as an infusion for sore throat. In the USP from 1820 to 1936 and in the National Formulary (NF) from 1936 to 1960, the plant was listed as an expectorant, cough remedy, emetic, and diuretic.

Wild cherry (*Prunus virginiana L.*)—The steeped bark can be taken as a tea for coughs and colds, and by some, also for lung trouble. The USP (1820–present) lists it as a sedative and pectoral and the syrup as a flavoring agent.

Tall cinquefoil (*Drymocallis arguta*)—This plant was used as a styptic to stop bleeding. Various species of puffballs also were used as hemostatics to stop bleeding or hemorrhaging.

Balm of Gilead (*Populus candicans Ait.*) and Balsam poplar (*Populus balsamifera L.*)—The buds were boiled in fat to make a salve. The ointment was placed in the nostrils to relieve congestion from colds, bronchitis, and other respiratory ailments. These were listed in the NF (1916–1965) for their use as a stimulant and expectorant. (Although the Balm of Gilead shares the same name as the biblical remedy, they are not the same.)

Blue Flag (*Iris versicolor L.*)—The root of this plant was steeped and used for colds, for lung trouble, and as a burn and sore dressing. In the USP (1820–1895) and the NF (1916–1942), the blue flag root was said to be a cathartic emetic and diuretic.

SHARING THE INFORMATION

One of the fundamental teachings of the Midewiwin was that no tree, bush, or herb was without use and that many, even those used mainly as food, had curative properties. Nevertheless, the extensive Mide pharmacopoeia was not shared by all members, at least not immediately. Instruction on the practice of medicine, with the identification and uses of a number of different therapeutic species, took place whenever an initiate advanced from one grade to the next.

In addition to these times of special instruction, a Mide curer might go to an older man or woman to buy additional knowledge. In the old days, a person would not share any facts about medicinal plants, even with a family member, without compensation, apparently for fear that information given freely would not be accorded the proper respect.

Names were rarely given to plants; rather, a fresh plant would be shown to someone seeking knowledge. In addition to those herbs that formed part of the secret Mide knowledge, each Chippewa household had its own supply of medicinal plants for common ailments. If these failed, a Mide specialist would be called in.

The part of the plant most commonly used was the root because it was considered to contain the greatest healing power, but stalks, leaves, and flowers were also used. Usually, these plant parts were dried for storage and pulverized for use. Mide curers might use only one plant for treatment or combine several. Some preparations included as many as 20 different species. Usually, a Mide doctor would collect, prepare, and store medicinal herbs for the entire season, sometimes traveling to distant places where certain species were known to grow in greater abundance than at home.

Birch trees (trees of the genus *Betula*), were highly valued in Native American medicine. Decoctions of various parts of the birch were used by native doctors for stomach cramps, as teas for postpartum tonics, as medicinal seasoners, as incense for people suffering from catarrh, to treat tuberculosis, and as stimulants, diuretics, astringents, parasiticides, antiseptics, and counterirritants.

As among other Native American peoples all over the Western Hemisphere, herbal remedies were often administered as enemas. The Chippewa apparatus consisted of a syringe made from a deer bladder, a small birch tray on which the syringe was laid, and two measures for the medicine, a larger one for adults and a smaller one for children. A carefully measured amount of the medicine was put into the bladder, and a short piece of hollow reed was tied in the opening by means of a strip of slippery elm bark. The reed, about an inch long, was used only once and then burned—remarkably similar to the single-use, disposable medical equipment used in modern Western medicine.

The principal medicine administered in this way was the inner bark of the common white birch that was scraped and steeped in water. An astringent decoction of the wood of the ash tree was also used. White ash, mountain ash, black ash, and red ash were also widely used.

Medicinal plants were treated with the greatest respect: Before taking one from the ground, a little hole would be dug beside it and an offering of tobacco placed in it. Meanwhile, the plant would be respectfully addressed with a little speech, thanking it for giving its curative powers for the benefit of the people. Tobacco would also be offered to trees, such as the chokecherry (*Prunus virginiana*) or wild black cherry (*Prunus serotina*), whose bark was to be used as a medicinal decoction.

Was every remedy effective? No. Was all treatment pragmatic, based on experiment and observation? No. Magic played its role, for example, in the use of plants both as internal medicine and as prophylactic charms. As elsewhere, including Europe from the time of the ancient Greeks to recent centuries, the so-called "doctrine of signatures" played a role in Chippewa plant herbal medicine—certain plants whose leaves or other parts resembled an afflicted organ were thought to be effective in restoring that organ to health.

If these proved to be of therapeutic value, it was by coincidence. Nevertheless, Mide curers achieved some remarkable cures with an extensive herbal pharmacopoeia based, in the absence of scientific knowledge of their active medicinal constituents, on observation and experimentation, reinforced by faith in the supernatural or spirit power the *manidos* invested in the natural environment for the benefit of human and animal life.

SYMBOLIC HEALING IN NAVAJO MEDICINE

The Navajo—or, as they prefer to be known, the *Diné*, meaning "People" or "True People"—practice a form of symbolic curing that aims to reestablish beauty and balance. Through chant and pictorial art, the Navajo re-create the world as it was in the beginning, when the Holy Ones, by defeating the monsters of disharmony, made the earth fit for human life. It has rightly been called one of the great healing systems of the world.

HOZHO

When the Diné speak of *hozho*—the desirable and the natural condition of the world—they mean health, beauty, and harmony. Roughly translatable as the "Beauty Path," *hozho* is the natural, desirable way of the world. Disturbance or lack of *hozho* means sickness, disharmony, and ugliness. *Hozho*, then, is the condition that must be restored whenever a person, a family, the community, or the natural environment has fallen out of balance. Sickness, of whatever kind, disrupts balance, within the self and between the afflicted individual and everything that makes up the social, natural, and spiritual environment: family, friends, the community, plants, animals, geologic features, and, most important, the vast array of spiritual forces that inhabit and enliven the Navajo universe. In consequence, Navajo medicine is directed not toward an afflicted organ or a specific symptom but toward reestablishing the equilibrium—the condition of *hozho*—that has been disrupted by pathology, be it physical, mental, or social.

The Diné have blessing and curing rites for virtually everything: physical or emotional sickness; a soldier leaving for, or returning from, war; animals; places such as houses; crops and livestock; and even starting a new business. For the Diné, making things right, restoring health, or putting the individual and the group back on the beauty way, involves both the literary and visual arts. Together they re-create the world when the twin sons of Mother Earth and Father Sky have battled and defeated the Monster Spirits that represented darkness, ugliness, evil, and disharmony, thereby readying the earth for its human inhabitants. It was the Holy Ones and the Hero Twins who gave the Diné the stories to be sung in the curing chants. They also instructed the Diné how to represent themselves, the Hero Twins, the Monsters (also called Enemy Gods), the sacred animals and plants, and all the other participants and events in the primordial dramas.

The sandpainting depicting the adventures of the ancient ones along with the words of the chant wipe away the boundaries between the now and the mythologic past. The patient for whom the ceremony was called is seated in the center of the painting so that he or she may absorb its healing power. At the same time the Holy Ones and the mythical events depicted in the painting draw out the disharmonious forces that caused the illness or imbalance.

To accomplish the rigorous requirements of the ceremonies takes years of instruction under knowledgeable elders. Some curing rituals extend over many days and nights, requiring the creation (and destruction once they have done their job) of 50 or more consecutive sandpaintings. There is an enormous amount of artistic and literary skill involved, including the expertise and intimate knowledge of content and meaning of the ancient stories.

Altogether, the complete repertoire of symbolic healing numbers some two dozen different chants, each with scores and even hundreds of songs, and a total of perhaps 500 specialized sandpaintings. For example, the Hail Chant, which counteracts illness caused by cold and frost, is one of the *shortest* in the extensive inventory of Diné curing chants, and yet it consists of more than 400 songs!

A curing chant may be requested by an individual who feels him- or herself (or, more often, is perceived by others) to be out of balance with the social, natural, and supernatural environment. Dreams can also be signs that a chant is required. The worst kind of dream would be one in which the dreamer encounters a *chindi*, the restless spirit or ghost of a dead person. In such a case, a "sing" or curing chant is definitely indicated, lest the dream turn out to be prophetic and the dreamer fall victim to the unpacified spirit. Illness, dispute, injury, a relative's death—all these and more can cause disruption of the essential equilibrium, a divergence from the Beauty Path, a loss of *hozho*.

Some chants are intended not to expel illness but to secure benefits, such as protection by the Holy Ones for a journey or some other enterprise fraught with peril. The Diné fear contact with the dead, and there are cases on record where veterans returning from war asked for curing chants to cleanse themselves and heal spirits disturbed by the sight of so much carnage. To determine the cause of the malady, a shaman must be consulted. These shamanic diagnosticians are different from the "singers" who do the curing ceremonies. They are not trained or taught as the singers are, but rather their powers of diagnosis often come to them unannounced. The diagnostician might simply start to tremble and go into a trance, performing a "handtremble" over the patient. While in the trance, they may trace various designs on the floor; these designs are interpreted later after the trancing. Once the cause had been divined, the diagnostician prescribes the appropriate chant to cure it. The patient or family engages the healer skilled in the proper songs and the accompanying artworks and provides the assistants that will help the specialist in the creation of the many different designs.

The curing takes place in a specially prepared and consecrated *hogan*, the traditional eight-sided Navajo dwelling similar to the yurts of central Asian and Siberian nomads. Offerings for the Holy Ones, including feathers, turquoise, tobacco, cornmeal, and other consecrated foodstuffs, are placed outside the *hogan* so that the ancestor spirits will see them and be pleased. The rituals of the first night are repeated on three successive nights, while the patient is instructed in the sacred lore, purified with steam baths, and given aromatic and medicinal herbs. There is always a prescribed order for the different actions of the curing drama; deviation can render them ineffective. The making of the first sandpainting does not begin until the fifth day. By nightfall it must be wiped away and its materials, which have soaked up the negative forces troubling the patient, returned to nature.

The making of these sacred designs is a marvel to behold. First the healer lays down a bed of light-colored sand. He holds the pigment in the palm of his hand and allows it to trickle out between his first and second fingers, using his thumb as a guide. For every change of color he cleans his hand by rubbing it with sand. The flat colors are laid down first, with details of costumes and accoutrements added in other colors, always working from large areas to small, and from the inside to the outside. Often the scene is encircled by a protective snake, or, more commonly, the elongated rainbow guardian. The sandpainting and chanting represent a kind of healing that is foreign to most modern non-indigenous Americans. It is mythical healing, in which the implications of illness and disease are grander than simply the symptoms of the illness.

In his book *Navajo Symbols of Healing*, Donald Sandner writes: "There is no question that often the time and resource necessary for a chant prevented or delayed the timely use of a specific, effective scientific remedy . . . If I had tuberculosis or appendicitis, or cancer in its early stages, I would be quick to avail myself of modern medicine. But if I had one of those maladies for which science has no specific cure, like cancer in its later stages or some psychiatric illness, I would prefer the symbolic healing of the Navajo."